W9-BNQ-088

YOU DON'T HAVE TO SUFFER

YOU DON'T HAVE TO SUFFER

A HANDBOOK FOR MOVING BEYOND LIFE'S CRISES

Judy Tatelbaum

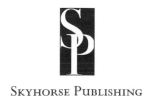

SKYHORSE PUBLISHING

Grateful acknowledgment is made to the following for permission to reprint selected material used as epigraphs at the opening of each chapter, including: David Schoenbrun. Reprinted by permission of the author and the author's agents, Scott Meredith Literary Agency, Inc., 845 Third Avenue, New York, New York 10022. *The Power of Positive Nonsense* Copyright © 1977 by Leo Rosten. Reprinted by permission of the author. *The Poetry of Robert Frost* edited by Edward Connery Lathem Copyright © 1934 by Holt, Rinehart and Winston and renewed 1962 by Robert Frost. Reprinted by permission of Henry Holt and Company, Inc. *The Prince of Tides* by Pat Conroy. Copyright © 1986 by Pat Conroy. Reprinted by permission of Houghton Mifflin Company. *The Medusa and the Snail* by Lewis Thomas. Copyright © 1974, 1975, 1976, 1977, 1978, 1979, by Lewis Thomas. All rights reserved. Reprinted by permission of Viking Penguin, Inc. *Getting Well Again* Copyright © 1978 by O. Carl Simonton and Stephanie Matthews-Simonton. All rights reserved. *Man and Superman* by George Bernard Shaw, reprinted with permission of The Society of Authors, London, on behalf of the Bernard Shaw Estate.

Copyright © 2012 by Judy Tatelbaum

All Rights Reserved. No part of this book may be reproduced in any manner without the express written consent of the publisher, except in the case of brief excerpts in critical reviews or articles. All inquiries should be addressed to Skyhorse Publishing, 307 West 36th Street, 11th Floor, New York, NY 10018.

Skyhorse Publishing books may be purchased in bulk at special discounts for sales promotion, corporate gifts, fund-raising, or educational purposes. Special editions can also be created to specifications. For details, contact the Special Sales Department, Skyhorse Publishing, 307 West 36th Street, 11th Floor, New York, NY 10018 or info@skyhorsepublishing.com.

Skyhorse® and Skyhorse Publishing® are registered trademarks of Skyhorse Publishing, Inc.®, a Delaware corporation.

Visit our website at www.skyhorsepublishing.com.

10 9 8 7 6 5 4 3 2 1

Library of Congress Cataloging-in-Publication Data is available on file.

ISBN: 978-1-62087-160-7

Printed in the United States of America

In honor of my parents,
Esther Beckler Tatelbaum (1907–1984)
Abraham J. Tatelbaum, M.D. (1907–1985)
and
In honor of my husband,
Allan G. Marcus

Author's Note

I have chosen to republish *You Don't Have to Suffer* because so many readers have found it to be a life-altering book. At one time or another, we all struggle with problems of love, loss, family, and health. This book is full of tools for facing and recovering from adversity. May it help free you to create a satisfying life.

Judy Tatelbaum

CONTENTS

FOREWORD

I have been using *You Don't Have to Suffer* as the text in my Mental/Emotional Health course at Northern Illinois University for close to twenty years. As an educator I wanted a resource that would supplement our discussions on an array of issues connected to emotional well being, such as understanding ourselves, life stages, control, needs, feelings, and how to bounce back when our lives are not going in the direction we would like.

As an educator I sought a text that conveyed information in a clear, easy to follow style. As a therapist I wanted that resource to provide direction and motivation for individuals in making changes in their lives. This was critical, since information by itself may not be enough to generate personal change.

I wanted my course to be one that would help students deal with the realities of their lives. Life is difficult. A happily ever after may not exist. Loved ones have died. Romantic relationships have ended. They have trust issues with the opposite sex. Dreams have been shattered. They have been abandoned by parents, and those with both parents realize they were not June and Ward Cleaver.

You Don't Have to Suffer is an engaging and refreshing book that provides direction and hope to readers. Judy's writing style invites readers to examine their lives in a fashion that encourages change and growth rather than suffering through life's disappointments. It is easy for individuals to relate to the examples presented. Strategies for change are provided in conjunction with Judy's thoughts on how we can make our lives work for us.

You Don't Have to Suffer has been a time-tested resource for me. My many students have gained great value from it. I am excited that a new edition is forthcoming and will continue to use what I feel is an excellent guide for living for many semesters to come.

Daniel Klein, PhD, MSW
School of Allied Health Professions
Public Health & Health Education
Northern Illinois University, DeKalb, Illinois

YOU DON'T HAVE TO SUFFER

But if a man happens to find himself . . . he has a mansion
which he can inhabit with dignity all the days of his life.

JAMES MICHENER

This book was inspired by a gift my mother gave me. In October 1984, knowing she was dying of cancer, my mother asked me not to cry for her. Filled with love, sorrow, and anguish, I said, "I can't promise you that. After all you are my mother . . . ." Her response was, "Okay, cry a little, but don't spend too much time on it."

In saying, "Don't cry for me," my mother opened up a possibility that had not existed for me before—the possibility of living the rest of my life not suffering over her death and maybe not suffering over any other of life's events. This was an extraordinary idea, considering that it took me fourteen years to recover from my brother's death. My mother's legacy to me was that she gave me a choice about whether or not to suffer. I am writing this book to pass her gift on to everyone who is open to her message: *You Don't Have to Suffer.*

I know I could have used this message earlier in my life, for I have dealt with much illness and death. I was involved with my parents' chronic illnesses during the last thirty years of their lives. Then in the five years after my book *The Courage to Grieve* was published, I experienced the sad endings of two love relationships and the deaths of five close friends from cancer: Tommy Berman, a wise friend and mentor since we were little children; Zoe Snyder, an exciting, beloved friend; Jim Simkin, my superb Gestalt therapy trainer, who loved me like a daughter; Al Parker, the fabulous illustrator, a loving supporter and "pretend" dad; and Lyn Friedman, a wonderful, supportive friend. These losses were followed by the deaths of both my parents within nine months of each other—my mother of cancer and then my father of heart disease complicated by grief.

I certainly have known suffering. And I am not suffering now. My choice: I could spend all the rest of my days sorrowing over all the loved ones I have lost, caught up in how bad the rough times have been, or I could let all that go and generate new loved ones, new satisfactions, new joys. I began writing this book two weeks after my father died as a statement to him and to me that I could create a life worth living with or without my family. Two years later, the week I finished the first draft of this book, I met my husband-to-be, certainly a result of my commitment not to suffer.

I have come to realize there is no limit to our ability to move and grow and change except within our own perceptions of what is possible. It became clear to me that time was not necessarily what it took to make changes or to heal, for in fact willingness and commitment play a much larger part in leading us to resolution or change. My psychotherapy work with people changed dramatically after that realization, and I was able to help people to more easily create whatever momentum they wanted or needed in their lives.

My most critical discoveries are that how we suffer and how much we suffer are very much our own choice, not a random experience, and that we can always transform ourselves from the experiences that hurt us. My intention with this book is to unmask the possibility for us that we do not have to suffer to the extent that we usually do, particularly in living through what might be thought of as catastrophic or poignant life experiences. Even though life may present us with a vast range of trying or difficult experiences or ordeals, we can choose how we respond to them and how we use them in our own development and expansion. Since satisfying lives are not our birthright, this book can also generate insights and tools for continually creating satisfying lives. More than we may ever wish to know, life is up to us. My message is *choose*: choose life, not suffering!

• How to Use This Book •

Having the Courage to Grow

Courage is grace under pressure.

Ernest Hemingway

Being fully alive to life is truly a heroic act. Being a conscious, responsible, and creative human being is living heroically. Many of us think heroism means rescuing people from burning buildings or being daring in wartime. Instead, heroism is an everyday affair. For some of us, getting up in the morning and facing another day is a heroic act. For others, changing jobs or staying in a relationship or managing to survive on limited funds or facing the loss of a loved one is a heroic act. We have many opportunities to be heroes in our daily lives. The heroism of which I speak is the courage to be fully alive to life regardless of our circumstances. This book is about generating that kind of courage in the face of the fact that life hurts.

If you use it as a guide, as a support, as a teacher, this book can be of enormous help. It can truly teach you how not to suffer. The tools are here. However, you cannot learn how to live from reading a book unless you put into action what you learn. Let the material come alive for you. Let it make a difference.

This book will be especially useful if you read it searching for understanding, validation, and openings for expanding your life. Read it with compassion for yourself. If you knew how to manage more easily and effectively, you would do it. Read with the understanding that each of us does the best we can at any moment.

The message of this book is about having power and control over your pain. The good news is that we can powerfully manage the difficult events in our lives, and the bad news is that we unwittingly create a great deal of our own misery. In the following chapters we will look at common behaviors that generate unhappiness. We will see how we exaggerate our pain when we personalize impersonal events, or dramatize, or live in the past. We will uncover how we cause our own suffering, and that we do not have to suffer anymore.

The ideas presented in this book will challenge you, relieve you, or perhaps disturb you. You need to be willing to be uncomfortable, for *You Don't Have to Suffer* may reveal unknown, unexpected, or startling features of yourself. Remember that it takes courage to be willing to uncover new or hidden aspects of ourselves. Such self-revelations can be exciting, uncomfortable, or even disturbing. Do not use these new insights to invalidate or judge or torture yourself. Indeed, allow them to stimulate and inspire you. Look for the new possibilities your insights can open up for you toward mastering your life, relieving suffering, and augmenting your ability to live truly satisfied. Know that you cannot help but grow and expand as a result of your new awareness.

Your willingness to experiment with or to try on new ideas will enhance your reading. See if the concepts fit for you. Allow this book to provoke you, consider what is said, evaluate, and use what is of value. You may want to reread particular sections for support in handling any uncomfortable or challenging moments that may lie ahead.

As you read, you may see that up to now you have been a victim of some entrenched and habitual behaviors of which you were unaware. In order to heal or expand, we need to know what we are doing that hurts or disempowers us and thus delays our healing. Undermining behaviors—such as romanticizing, personalizing, and living in the past—will be addressed first, and later you will see particular areas in life where most of us get "stuck": separation, grief, parents, and our health. *You Don't Have to Suffer* concludes with many suggestions for overcoming suffering, with emphasis on forgiving, completing, and healing yourself.

One way to read this book would be to have a notebook alongside to jot down your realizations or your plans for future actions. You can experiment with the many exercises throughout the book. Some readers have suggested using this book as a kind of workbook for personal problem solving. It is up to you to use whatever techniques in reading that would benefit you the most.

The secret of living well is not in the answers we amass but in the actions we take. Read this book knowing that it does not contain the definitive or "right" answers to life. Although we all hunger for them, there are no surefire answers that will make much of a difference in the quality of our lives. Underlying our wish for answers or solutions is the illusion that life should be problem free. No matter how many problems we solve, there will always be new ones to take their place. We can be more masterful in life if we allow problems to be an ever-present, challenging, and stimulating aspect of living.

Open yourselves to new discoveries by reading this book with a profound appreciation for who you are and who you can be. Even if you do nothing new, *You Don't Have to Suffer* can provide you with solace and compassion for yourself. You will see that our experiences and feelings are universal, no matter how bewildering or peculiar or different we may privately think they are. Accepting and embracing our own humanity is one of the secrets of living life truly satisfied and free of suffering.

This book cannot be about the end of suffering. Rather, it is about discovering satisfaction even in the wake of suffering. It is about living fully, living with power, dignity, and creativity, regardless of your particular circumstances and all the limitations implicit in humanness and human experience. It is about learning to transcend our circumstances and those beliefs and ideas that limit us. It is about completing the past, so that we are always free to move forward.

The purpose of *You Don't Have to Suffer* is to stimulate and inspire you to approach life with a greater commitment to satisfaction than to suffering. This can be an awesome task because of the vast opportunities and experiences we confront. At every moment we get to choose whether to live fully awake and alive to life or closed down and suffering. We are often unaware that how we live is our choice. My wish is that from now on you will choose how you live and, out of choosing, that you will see your power to transform any and all of your experiences.

> *Except for those who have given permission to appear in this book, all names and identifying details of individuals mentioned in this book have been changed. In some instances, composite accounts have been created based on the author's professional expertise.*

•I•

WE CAN CHOOSE NOT TO SUFFER

•1•

HURT IS INEVITABLE—
SUFFERING IS NOT

A hero is no braver than an ordinary man,
but he is braver five minutes longer.

RALPH WALDO EMERSON

Life hurts. Fate throws us many different kinds of curves. In a full life we are presented with tough tests: crises and obstacles, pain and hardships, failures and tragedies. For all of us, the journey through life is full of changes and surprises. Few of us find the way to be smooth and easy. How we experience our own journey is up to us, for we can choose to view life either as a challenge and an opportunity or as a predicament.

We hurt. The human heart is very sensitive. It is natural to feel sad, to be angry, disappointed, or discouraged. The problem is not that we hurt, but that our hurt continues so long after events occur. Suffering is extended hurt. Suffering is the persistence of painful feelings long after they were provoked. Just because suffering is common among us does not mean that it is necessary, and yet we often suffer because we do not know what else to do.

We perpetuate our own suffering. Although we usually believe that our circumstances, such as our tragedies or disappointments, cause our suffering, that is not true. Suffering is not implicit in circumstances, any kind of circumstances, but rather in the way we view and respond to the circumstances in our lives. This is evident in how different people react to similar events, as not every one of us suffers or responds identically.

One friend who lost all her belongings in a fire was desolate and inconsolable for months, while another seemed quite at ease with her loss, saying she felt "free of history," free to create her life anew.

One patient with cancer was devastated and felt hopeless. Another began helping other patients as they sat together waiting for their daily chemotherapy.

Two sets of parents in one of my workshops had each lost a teenaged daughter. One couple, whose daughter was murdered, was determined to recover and go on with their lives. The other couple, whose daughter died in an accident, kept saying they would "never recover," and nothing could in any way console them.

The ending of a marriage can be profoundly painful, and still we see many kinds of reactions to separation or divorce. Usually divorce is an ordeal. Couples may be angry, hurt, even devastated. They may express their pain or hide their feelings. Some ex-spouses grieve for months, even years, and find it hard to establish a new lifestyle alone. Others take the opportunity of newfound freedom to create a new, more satisfying life on their own or with a new partner. Although every relationship's ending has a unique quality, we can see that it is not the circumstance of divorce that causes our suffering, but how we each respond or react to it.

My friend Jan is an inspiration. A few months after her husband left her, she introduced me to her new lover. Startled at Jan's quick passage from one relationship to another, I asked her about the speed with which she mastered her grief and began with someone new. She laughed and said, "I guess I just don't like to suffer." Unlike Jan, many of us think we must suffer, that it is a necessary and unavoidable part of life. As Jan demonstrates, we can finish quickly with painful events if we choose.

Though we may not always be able to avoid pain, we can choose how much we suffer. Unfortunately, we often feel powerless over our suffering. Thinking we have no other choice, we get "stuck" in pain and stay there much too long. Suffering becomes a habit. We get used to wearing mourning clothes or telling the story of our tragedy, used to feeling upset, sad, or lonely. Thus we just continue to live in misery as if that is our only choice. But it is possible to stop extending that misery.

We do not have to prolong suffering. We certainly do not have to spend our whole lives in pain. We can control some of the ways we suffer, the amount of time we allot to it, and the depth of our discomfort. We can ask ourselves, "How long am I going to take to handle and recover from this event?" We can set a time limit, rather than waiting and hoping for our distress to diminish magically or disappear of its own accord. I met a woman who had grieved twenty-seven years over her mother's death, proving we can grieve forever if we don't stop ourselves. We have to take responsibility for ending our own suffering.

We don't even have to view our experiences as painful or trying. We can control the extent of our suffering by how we view what happens to us. Accepting death as inevitable rather than seeing it as an incomprehensible event, a personal punishment, or a terrible deprivation, for example, lessens the blow of losing a loved one. Accepting loss, change, illness, and accidents as parts of a full life, not as devastating events from which we cannot recover, makes them easier to face.

Consider four people who had polio and chose different ways to deal with it: The first was angry all the time, believing this disease had ruined her life; the second, navigating on crutches, was outwardly independent yet subtly whiny and pathetic; the third seemed at ease with and unaffected by his disability; and the last, Franklin Roosevelt, was a great leader and innovator despite the limitations of his body. Although they may not have consciously chosen their responses to polio, we can see that these four people coped with a traumatic illness in very different ways.

We must realize that we always have a choice to make, a serious and conscious choice, as to how we will react to distressing life events. It may be hard to admit that we create our own suffering in response to our circumstances. Yet that admission gives us the power to choose our responses instead of just letting our circumstances direct or control us.

We really don't have to suffer, unless we choose to do so. Yet to simply stop suffering is a radical idea that challenges our beliefs and behaviors. Although we long to be contented and satisfied, the idea of living free of pain or unhappiness may seem unfathomable. Thus, we must unravel the beliefs that keep us suffering.

Suffering is not a prerequisite for happiness. Yet many of us believe that suffering is necessary and even noble. We may think we are "better" people for having suffered. We aren't. We do not have to suffer in order to grow or learn. We do not have to suffer to gain life's rewards. We do not have to suffer to become enlightened.

However, we can use powerful circumstances as stepping stones to our growth. Instead of just perpetuating our misery, we can choose to use any circumstances, even the terrible events or anguished moments, to develop wisdom, to alter our lives, and perhaps to contribute in some way to the world.

We can alter our relationship with suffering. By examining the ways we stop ourselves from successfully moving through life's challenges, we can learn to move beyond each crisis or disappointment. We can allow the experience and then just let it go. We can learn to transcend our circumstances, terrible or painful though they may be. Transcending our circumstances, rather than perpetually suffering over them, is one of the major secrets of living a full and satisfying life.

We can learn to broaden our abilities and to expand our repertoire for coping with the ordeals and opportunities life presents to us. To do so will take courage—the courage to live fully, consciously, and responsibly. For some of us, courage would seem an inappropriate word to describe how we have played out our lives up to now. Yet changing our ways invariably takes enormous courage—the courage to change and perhaps admit that we were wrong, the courage to confront whatever is the truth about ourselves and our lives, the courage to experiment and learn and be awkward, and the courage to be fully, uniquely who we are, alive and engaged in life.

Most of all, we need the courage to face the hurts of life. Since suffering is hurt that has been prolonged, we need to come to terms with and accept the inevitability of being hurt.

• 2 •

ACCEPTING THAT LIFE HURTS

The game of life is not so much in holding a good hand
as playing a poor hand well.

H. T. LESLIE

Hurt is a fact of life. Until we accept and allow that hurt is inevitable, we cannot begin to deal more effectively with the hurts of life. As human beings, we will hurt and be hurt. None of us is invulnerable. Not only do circumstances upset us, but we hurt each other, not necessarily intentionally or maliciously. We disappoint, criticize, anger, injure, and withhold from one another all the time.

Because we refuse to accept and include hurt and the suffering that may follow as an inevitable aspect of human experience, hurt takes us by surprise and we never learn effective ways to deal with it. It is not wrong to hurt, but it is tragic that we let our reactions to hurt and our fear of hurt run our lives.

We hold hurt as wrong. We think that hurt should simply not happen to us. We imagine if we were good enough or mature enough or strong enough we would not hurt. In longing to be superhuman—not human—we deny the inevitability of hurting and being hurt. As a result we are outraged and often overwhelmed when we are hurt or disappointed.

If we only accepted that hurts happen, we would be much more effective in dealing with them. Then we could freely admit to inflicting or feeling hurt. With such a consciousness, we could simply recoil momentarily from pain and not feel damaged by every hurtful event in our lives. We would certainly be freer to forgive and forget, the most powerful way we can overcome hurt.

However, it is when we don't let hurt go that the results are tragic. We allow hurt to influence us very deeply, sometimes for the rest of our lives. Because we often believe that the past damage done to is irreparable, we allow hurts to color our future, often disadvantageously. We act in self-defeating ways to protect ourselves. We make stringent rules about how we are going to respond to people and relationships from now on, and these self-imposed rules may have an impact on the rest of our lives. Our rules often begin with the words, "I will never again." Then we do things like never again loving or giving or sharing ourselves intimately or asking for anything. Unknowingly, one single hurtful incident can become the basis for how we operate all the rest of our lives.

As a youngster, James was so hurt by his mother's withdrawal from him to take care of her three younger children that he vowed "never again to trust women, never again to love." Always alone, he lives virtually as a hermit, doing research and growing African violets.

Risa was so hurt by her husband's anger at her early in their marriage that she is now frozen in her responses to him, unable to share her feelings or to participate in sex with any satisfaction, and yet too frightened to leave and face more hurt in the world.

Once hurt, we simply write off aspects of living and our own aliveness from then on. Out of an experience of hurt we may suppress or withhold a part of ourselves. We may become very careful of how familiar or expressive or trusting we are; worse, we may not trust people again—period. We often make decisions that have an impact on us for years based on one hurtful moment, decisions that become our own destructive, self-fulfilling prophesies.

We are so afraid we will be hurt again, and we probably will be. Rather than living our lives based on fear of hurt or pain, preventing ourselves from having love and enjoyment, spontaneity and vitality, we need to learn to cope better with hurt. We cannot hide from it.

Few of us handle emotional hurt as masterfully as we handle physical hurt. If we bump our knee on the corner of a table, we might yelp or yell out and briefly be very aware of the pain. We might stop and rub that knee and feel sorry for ourselves for a moment. Then, the pain is over for us. Even though we may occasionally notice an ache or pain in that knee or remember our carelessness, the incident of the bruised knee is completed quickly and easily with a minimum of blame, shame, drama, or distress.

This is vastly different from how we usually handle emotional hurt. We don't punish our knees for causing physical pain. However, we do punish ourselves and other people for causing us emotional pain by rejecting others or withholding ourselves. This is neither an effective way to handle pain nor much protection against further hurt. In being cut off from intimacy and nourishment this way, we hurt ourselves.

But there is a way out. We can confront hurt and let it go. We can live full and intimate lives, allowing that we might be hurt occasionally. All it would take is for us to be able to say "Ouch!" or "That hurt!" to one another at appropriate moments, to express the pain and let it go. We do not have to suppress our feelings, for we can let them go more quickly. We cannot over-come the fact of hurt in life, and we can overcome our difficulties in coping with hurt—if we are willing.

Knowing now that we have a choice about how we approach hurt and suffering, we will look next at what it takes to make such a choice. At this point we may feel stirred up or confused, for the idea that we have any choice over hurt and suffering may challenge lifelong beliefs. Many of us have inadvertently lived as victims of our circumstances and our feelings for most of our lives. The next chapter, "Designing Our Destinies: Victims or Choosers," addresses that issue. We do not have to be victims any longer.

·3·

DESIGNING OUR DESTINIES: VICTIMS OR CHOOSERS

If I had my life to live over . . . I'd dare to make more mistakes
next time. I'd relax. I would limber up. I would be sillier
than I have been this trip. I would take fewer things
seriously. I would take more chances. I would take more trips.
I would climb more mountains and swim more rivers.
I would eat more ice cream and less beans . . .

NADINE STAIR, 85 YEARS OLD,
LOUISVILLE, KENTUCKY

Imagine what it could mean to us if we were willing to design our own destinies. We could be thrown a curve by life and not be thrown off course. We could recover quickly from a relationship's ending. We could lovingly let loved ones die and go on with our lives. We could lose property and not miss it. We could face the crisis of not having money or of losing a job and go on. We could take on and handle whatever life presented us, even the seemingly most unmanageable of life's events. People do. I have met people who survived disease, disaster, and tragic losses who are living full lives nonetheless. This is possible when we take charge of our lives, when we act as the power behind our lives instead of as the victims of our lives.

WE CAN BE VICTIMIZED BY NOT BEING RESPONSIBLE

When we don't take charge, we live as if we are a victim, often a helpless victim. Events and circumstances just happen to us. Disappointments, losses, illnesses, failures, accidents, and hardships seem to occur without our being prepared and seem to be out of our control. Sometimes it feels as if life bombards us with one crisis after another. Once confronted, we are either bowled over or we somehow muddle through. But we don't feel like we have much power or much choice in how we experience life. Thrown off by whatever occurs, we live afraid, hunched over, awaiting the next blow. If we stopped being so cautious and refused to play the victim, we would be freer to enjoy life and to take life on, no matter what might happen next.

Taking responsibility, taking on ownership of our lives, is the powerful alternative to being a victim. This means allowing, accepting, and participating in what happens to us, rather than resisting life's events. From the vantage point of ownership, we can look for what we can learn, how we can grow, and how we can ultimately make our lives more rewarding as a result of any experience.

When we are living responsibly, we can create value out of our experiences. Then an illness or the breakup of a relationship can be a useful stopping place to reexamine life, to weed out what is unimportant and to nurture that which has meaning to us. An accident could be a time for appreciating what we have and almost lost. A failure could be a chance to generate new goals or to develop more skills. Most important, instead of considering ourselves the victim of an accident or crisis, we could include it as one of the many experiences offered us in a full lifetime.

We do not cause tragic events. Responsibility for and ownership of our lives does not mean seeing ourselves as the cause of the events or circumstances in our lives, for we do not have the power to cause earthquakes or tornadoes, to make other people live or die or be happy or sad.

Instead, being responsible means taking charge of how we respond to or handle our reactions. Our power over our lives comes from how we confront life's challenges. Ownership of our reactions can potently alter our experience of our circumstances. Even if we have no control over many of the events that occur in life, we can have some control over ourselves. We are most powerful when we take life on, face it, learn from it, let it go, and go on anew, while as victims we can only be overwhelmed, powerless, "stuck."

Richard's mother was injured and his sister died in a house fire. At first he felt helpless and thought of running away, but he realized how much his mother needed him. He saw that he had a choice, and he chose to manage this tragedy instead of succumbing to it. He flew to his mother's side and managed all the details of the funeral, his mother's injuries, and finding her a temporary new home. We would all understand if Richard had been immobilized in coping with this misfortune, yet he told me later he couldn't give in to feeling helpless with his family in such great need. He chose not to be a victim of those terrible events. As a result, he was less consumed with grief and felt enormous self-respect. Applying this to any life circumstance, we can see how powerful choosing can be.

WE CAN BE VICTIMIZED BY OUR REACTIONS

What usually leads us to feel without choice, out of control in life, are our automatic reactions to events or experiences: reactions like fear, anxiety, defensiveness, anger, sadness, guilt, and disappointment, to name a few. All of us react. We suddenly become upset or defensive when we think we have been criticized or maligned. We automatically become angry when someone tells us what to do. We feel a rush of fear when it is our turn to stand and speak. We blush with shame when someone tells us we made a mistake. Our hearts beat rapidly when we hear bad news.

It is not the circumstances that make us hurt; it is our own reactions to them. Events occur and we react. For most of us, reactions simply happen to us or in us. We have no sense that they are either separate from us or in our control, so we feel like victims of our reactions. Usually we blame life's events or crises for being the cause of our distress, when really our distress is the result of our responses to those events.

We can choose to be more powerful than our feelings and thoughts, even if we believe we have no choice in regard to our reactions. Rather than being dominated by feelings we can, for instance, feel the blush of embarrassment (or anger), notice it, admit we are embarrassed, then let it go, take our attention off it, and go on. We do not have to be stopped by this feeling. Richard felt helpless and took action in spite of that. This holds true whether we are anxiously anticipating an upsetting scenario or feeling distressed about an event that has already occurred. Whenever we notice any reaction, we can acknowledge that feeling or thought, and then we can stop paying attention to it. It is up to us, our choice, whether we embrace our feelings and thoughts (our reactions) or release them.

Until now we may not have known we have any choice about how we react. This discovery was made poignantly clear to me several years ago when my lifelong friend Tommy Berman called and said, "I have something to tell you, and I don't want you to react emotionally to it." Then he told me he had brain cancer and probably six months to live. I gulped, swallowed, and went on talking with him naturally, much as if we were discussing his having a cold. Tommy set the stage so well for us that we were always able to talk frankly about his disease and his impending death. (Our honesty also helped me to accept his death when the time came.) In honoring his request not to react emotionally, I was able to be involved and honest with Tommy, rather than avoiding him or being overwhelmed by the facts or my grief, fear, or anger. Tommy taught me a very important lesson. We can choose to manage our own reactions under any circumstances.

Oftentimes a feeling, any feeling, takes precedence over everything else, for we tend to be swept up by and to embrace any feeling or thought that comes our way. We automatically give weight and attention to our feelings. Yet if we do not hold on to them, feelings and thoughts naturally just come and go, like clouds that pass regularly through the sky. However, when we don't see that we are separate from our feelings, we feel overwhelmed by them. In reaction to this, some of us have learned to suppress our feelings, but this doesn't help us cope or resolve anything, either.

Our power is in allowing feelings but not hanging on to them. I am not proposing stifling or denying our feelings. I am proposing that the secret of getting through painful experiences quickly and easily is in living them moment to moment. This means feeling pain when we feel pain and then letting it go, being angry when we are angry and then letting it go, and the same with any of our feelings.

WE CAN BE VICTIMIZED BY OUR BELIEFS

Until now, we may not have realized the extent to which our lives are both affected by and designed by our beliefs, often unconscious beliefs. We are apt to be victims of our beliefs unless we make them conscious. Once uncovered, beliefs are simply a set of ideas or convictions that we accept as true. In other words, we empower our own beliefs, and we make them true. Thus if we believe something will hurt us, it probably will. If we believe we will always feel a certain way, we will. This is particularly significant and tragic when we believe we will always grieve. Then no matter what we learn to the contrary, we are apt to honor that belief and grieve always.

Destructive beliefs: At times our beliefs can be a real detriment to us. When we believe we are victims of or chosen for life's tragedies, we feel powerless to intervene or to heal. When we believe that suffering makes us noble or better than other people, we are apt to suffer, no matter what. If we believe we cannot manage our emotions, chances are they can be overwhelming. Even if we are unaware of them, these kinds of destructive beliefs deeply influence our lives and victimize us.

Constructive beliefs: On the other hand, when our beliefs support us, they greatly enhance our lives. The belief that we can accomplish anything, or the belief that we are guided by some higher power, or the belief that everything that happens to us enhances our growth: all of these cause wonderful results.

Even when healing might have looked impossible to accomplish, when we believe we can heal, we are more likely to do so. My father had severe heart disease beginning at the age of forty-seven. He believed he could live with very faulty arteries to his heart and he lived to age seventy-eight.

When we believe we can recover from emotional hurts, we invariably do. I met a couple who lost twins as a result of congenital problems shortly after birth. This couple was an inspiration because they accepted this painful experience as a necessary part of their own maturity. They believed that they would grow best from letting go and living fully without grief. As a result, they generated satisfying and fulfilling lives, and they ultimately had another child.

DISCOVERING OUR BELIEFS

Since our destructive beliefs get us into the most trouble, we need a means for managing them. Uncovering faulty beliefs can be done simply by asking ourselves in any situation, "What beliefs do I have about this?" We should write those beliefs down. Then we have them concretely in front of us to see and evaluate. Once beliefs are revealed, we have a choice about them. We are no longer influenced without our knowledge.

Here are kinds of victimizing beliefs:

I can't
We can't change how we are
We cannot recover
We never get over a loss
Today will always be the same as yesterday
If we hurt, we will always hurt
If we loved someone, we must grieve forever to prove our love

All of us are filled with all kinds of beliefs about everything in life, beliefs that have mostly lived unexamined within us. Any time is an opportunity to discover our beliefs and to see whether or not those beliefs are beneficial and life-enhancing. The different topics throughout this book present opportunities for uncovering and examining our beliefs. Let's remember that our power over our reactions and our beliefs lies in owning that we are in charge here. Thus we can alter or design our beliefs to support our lives. Becoming aware is the first step.

DESIGNING OUR DESTINY

It is natural to be reluctant to face the difficulties or crises in our lives. We know that if we had anything to do with writing the story of our lives, we would not have let this event happen or this person disturb us. Take another perspective: What if we actually did select this event from the myriad of experiences because of the good it would do us, or the growth that would result, or the difference it would make for someone else? We shouldn't clobber ourselves with this idea, but play with it.

Years after my brother's death, I realized that much of my psychotherapy practice involved grief work. If I had not had that trauma, I might never have been able to help all those people. Although I did not consciously choose to have that tragedy, it turned out that the worst thing that happened in my life did benefit me and a lot of other people as well.

It is paradoxical that what truly makes life sing for us is change, and yet change is what we most dread and fear. What if we welcomed the changes wrought by our confrontations with life? What if we saw them as powerful stepping stones to our growth and maturity? Welcoming life instead of resisting it, hating it, or fearing it might be our single greatest source of power in coping with it. Welcoming life allows us to be the chooser, the designer of our own destiny. In a similar vein, choosing between viewing life as a predicament or as a challenge is addressed in the next chapter, "Choosing to Transform Painful Experiences: Life as a Challenge or a Predicament."

•4•

CHOOSING TO TRANSFORM PAINFUL EXPERIENCES: LIFE AS A CHALLENGE OR A PREDICAMENT

Whatever you can do or dream you can, begin it.
Boldness has genius, power, and magic in it.

GOETHE, *FAUST*

What is extraordinary about us is that we each have the capacity to rise like the phoenix out of our own ashes, to create ourselves anew, to begin again. We can transform ourselves and our lives, regardless of what we have endured before now. Maybe the true purpose of suffering is that out of our pain we will rise, expand, grow, and achieve.

We each have an amazing and powerful capability for insight and change. We can awaken, enlighten ourselves, shift our view or our behavior, and turn our lives around. That is transformation. When we grasp our power to transform, we have the proverbial "keys to the kingdom." Even though these "keys" are available to everyone, most of us never get to use them. Instead, we keep ourselves victims entrenched in suffering because of beliefs that we may not even be aware of and because of fear or unwillingness to change. The road to transformation can be filled with many potential pitfalls.

Seeing the opportunity instead of the predicament in distressing events is one way to empower ourselves and to transform our suffering. It is interesting that the Chinese use the same character for crisis and for opportunity. We would be less apt to consider ourselves victims if we saw that the events that provoke our suffering also offer us the opportunity to expand our ideas, awareness, actions, and aliveness. In a crisis we discover our ability to confront and survive life's challenges, and from a crisis we can mature, transforming ourselves and our lives. The ability to transform our experiences, reactions, or confrontations with life turns all of life into an opportunity.

Seeing the opportunity in suffering can be difficult, for it is natural to neither want pain nor see any redeeming value in it. When we are right in the midst of the suffering, in the midst of grief, anguish, or distress, which one of us can see any purpose in it? I have never sat in the middle of a painful moment and thought it was worth it. However, it would be very powerful if we each could say, this is the hand I have been dealt; now I'll play it as well as I can.

Usually it is only when a particular trauma is over or when the pain ceases that we look back and know that we were altered, even transformed, by the hurt, disappointment, or tragedy. Then we can see how we approached, handled, or experienced something differently than ever before.

Transformation is a spontaneous shift in our perspective or behavior, a shift in how we see our experience, or a sudden shift in how we act. Although we may not address it as such, all of us have experienced transformation in our everyday lives, those times when our actions or feelings or viewpoint altered suddenly. After we let go of an old anger or hurt, all at once a relationship feels new and different. We are transformed when we do not get angry at the same old thing, when we do a task or handle a problem in a new way, or when we take some action that we never thought we could take.

Out of fear and a deep sense of inadequacy, Louise dreaded ever having to handle any family crisis, but when she gave birth to a handicapped child, she amazed people with her courage and her ability to handle a difficult situation with ease. She told me that she saw that this child really needed her, so "I simply did it. I was totally different than I thought I would be, and now I know how capable I am."

We can transform ourselves or our lives, even if we don't believe we can. We may think transformation is a magical occurrence, like a bolt from the blue. Transformation is not magic, even though sometimes our shifts seem magical. Just as we often feel that we are victims, that hardships just happen to us, we may think transformation just happens to us, too. However, through awareness, willingness, action, and commitment, we have the ability to direct our own transformation.

People amaze me with their creativity in coping with and resolving what seem to be the most terrible of life's offerings. Choosing to see life as a challenge instead of as a predicament is one way people transform painful experiences. The following are several examples of individuals who transformed traumatic events into foundations for their growth and achievement. Let these people serve as inspiration to use painful experiences to move forward in some powerful new way.

Legally blind, Marybeth became a champion skier and led other blind people on skiing trips. I told her that out of a fear of hurting myself, I had never even dared to ski. I asked her how she had found the courage to do this. She laughed and said, "I guess we blind people have less to worry about; we can't see anything." Marybeth was not held back by our common view of blindness as a limitation.

Sara and Rob were traveling when fire swept through the Santa Cruz Mountains and burned their home to the ground. They came home to find nothing left of their possessions. In the aftermath, friends commented on Sara's serenity and beauty, characteristics that they found bewildering in someone who had just lost everything she owned. Sara said that after a few days she had realized that "we were free of our history, free of the past." With that discovery she noticed she felt relieved, happier, and more creative than she had in years.

We recontextualize events when we shift our view. Sara shifted how she might ordinarily have viewed losing all her belongings in a fire. Instead of seeing it as a horrendous loss, a tragedy, she saw that she was experiencing freedom and relief. She recontextualized the fire from a tragedy to a new freedom for living, just as Marybeth altered her idea of her own potential by not maintaining the commonly held belief that blindness is limiting.

Our willingness to look at our lives from a new perspective opens the possibility of transformation. Roger lost the only copy of his doctoral thesis in a fire. Instead of being upset by the irreparable loss of his thesis, he welcomed the idea of creating new work. Maria lost her infant son as a result of SIDS—sudden infant death syndrome. She managed her loss philosophically, saying that it must not have been his time to live a full life. As a result, she did not blame herself or stay enmeshed for long in grief.

Another powerful example of transformation was Terry Fox, a young Canadian man who contracted bone cancer in both legs. His lower legs were removed and replaced by metal braces. Unstoppable, Terry ran on his metal legs across Canada to show support for ending hunger in the world. He took his attention off himself and his serious medical situation in order to have his life make a difference for others. It has. Taking a stand is a very powerful way of newly designing our lives. We take just as powerful a stand when we simply shift from "I can't" to "I can."

Many cancer patients have called cancer "a transformational disease" because of new possibilities that emerge during their life-and-death confrontation with it. In my work, I have seen phenomenal shifts in people after they are diagnosed as having cancer. Alice created a new level of sharing and intimacy with her husband. This was amazing because for years prior to her disease they lived in separate parts of their house, merely coexisting and not communicating. Katherine, an overly protective mother diagnosed with cancer, taught her three teenagers to manage their lives effectively. All three became outstanding achievers following her death.

Facing bodily injury, pain, or disfigurement can be a major trauma. Several years ago Miriam was in a serious automobile accident in which her whole body was burned. Over the next several years she had plastic surgery over her entire body, and she still remained scarred. As a result, Miriam has become an expert in the use of "camouflage" makeup and tattooing to help people like herself deal with their scars.

In *The Courage to Grieve* I gave several examples of individuals who transformed their lives after the deaths of loved ones. Afterward, I received many telephone calls and letters from people sharing poetry and books they had written and work they were doing with hospices and bereavement groups. Many of us have learned to make great contributions out of our sorrows, transforming our pain into valuable actions. Life is not only easier but more deeply satisfying when we take life as an opportunity instead of a torture or a predicament.

To insure that we make the kind of changes that we intend to make, that we transform our relationship with hurt and suffering, we may need to take a stand on ourselves and our lives, to commit ourselves to a new way of being. The next chapter addresses "The Commitment Not to Suffer."

• 5 •

THE COMMITMENT NOT
TO SUFFER

> *... The moment one definitely commits oneself,*
> *then providence moves too.*
>
> GOETHE, *FAUST*

Knowing now that we can choose not to suffer, one of the strongest ways to overcome suffering is to commit ourselves to stopping it. Taking this stand represents our willingness to forgo our distress and to be complete. It does not mean we are unfeeling or uncaring.

Giving our word and standing by our word, we can do anything, even stop suffering. A commitment is a stand we take that we will create or cause a change to actually occur, that we will affect our lives, not merely that we hope to effect a change in our lives. Committing ourselves means keeping our word day after day, and this commitment provides us with a structure from which to manage our lives.

Actually, we make these kinds of commitments to act or to control our lives all the time. Because we usually are not conscious of these promises, we may not realize we made them. As stated earlier, we frequently say, "I'll never _____ again," and live by it, as a self-fulfilling prophesy, often to our own detriment. We say we will never love again or never trust again. We say we will never again climb mountains or go dancing or eat Chinese food or see some troublesome person. Because we do this often and offhandedly, we don't see the power in such declarations. Nonetheless, our "never again" statements profoundly influence our lives.

"I will" is as powerful to say as "I won't." Spoken consciously, "I will" can have a profoundly positive effect on our lives. Declaring that we will do something, even something as incredible as "I will stop suffering," can benefit us beyond our wildest dreams. We can declare, "I will never again suffer," or "I will never again blame my husband," or "I will never again put myself down," or "I will never complain."

Saying these words once, of course, is not enough, but making these declarations as a daily reminder of the life-style change that is being implemented can be very effective. When traveling with friends last year, we all promised each other not to complain. It began as a promise not to complain about the hot weather. Then we experimented with no complaining, period. Reminding myself not to complain helped me overcome all kinds of obstacles. As a result, I have never enjoyed a trip more or managed the unpleasant aspects of traveling better—the crowds, changes in schedules, long hours of driving, difficult people, and unfamiliarity with the language.

When we are intent on overcoming hurt or suffering, we may need to take some preliminary steps before we promise to draw those feelings to a close. We may first need to release or express our emotions and reactions related to the upsetting experience. We have strong feelings and reactions in response to painful moments in life. Being aware of our feelings may not be enough, for to shortcut pain we may need to voice our sadness, fears, longings, regrets, angers, or whatever it is we are feeling. This means speak now, not waiting for next week or next year or a better time to release—perhaps forever—all that is connected with this painful moment. Our feelings can dissolve and disappear whenever we express ourselves fully.

We must be willing to forgive and forget, to let go of our pain and go on. This is where many of us are unpracticed, for we habitually carry everything that has happened to us around in an ever-present storage bin called "the story of our life." Nothing keeps pain alive more than remembering it, so learning to forgive and forget is essential. Remember, suffering is perpetuating the pain of the past and carrying it into the future.

Dee quit a prestigious job to stay home for several months to take care of her ill husband. After she had expressed her grief in therapy, I suggested that she did not have to suffer further over these drastic changes in her life. Dee promised to stop suffering, and then consciously made this new experience a challenge to enjoy. She read a lot and learned to cook in a new, more healthy way. Ultimately she found that she enjoyed taking care of her husband, and their relationship was richer for it. Keeping her commitment not to suffer made a big difference.

What is so powerful is that we can actually commit ourselves in advance to be any way we want to be. We can commit ourselves not to suffer or not to agonize over a disappointment. We can commit to be satisfied with life or to be complete with whatever has occurred, to live effortlessly instead of struggling, to be free of worry or free of the past. This is clearly a potent means for shifting our attitudes or behaviors. Our promises give us power; they release us from the idea that we are victims of anything.

When I told her about the possibility of promising not to suffer, Barbara stopped agonizing over her son's leaving home and going to college. Instead, she got busy with new enlivening activities.

When Lee committed herself to stop suffering over being ill and missing three months of work, she felt relieved and happier than she had in a long time.

Several clients successfully ended their extended suffering over relationships that broke up. One woman took a stand that she would handle her divorce with dignity and did so. A man stopped upsetting himself about the financial cost of his divorce and freed himself of lifelong concerns about money.

On my last visit to my father after my mother died, my father was in despair, wondering why he was still alive with such severe heart problems and grief. He did not want to live without my mother. I said, "Daddy, I don't know why you are still alive, but I'm glad you and Mom didn't die at the same time. I couldn't have handled that then. Now, I can. I want you to know I am a competent grown-up, and as much as I hate to lose you, I can take it." My father died three days later.

I committed myself ahead of time to a very powerful stand when I told my father in advance of his death that "I can take it." It wasn't that I knew I could. I didn't know. I made it up to assure myself that I could. Even though I was now confronting something I had dreaded and feared for years, the deaths of my parents, my stand supported me to go on with my life. By declaring myself able, I was not overwhelmed by grief. To keep that promise, I began writing this book two weeks after my father died. I engaged myself in a new, involving project to ensure that I would keep my word. My experience with my father demonstrates that we can take a stand to overcome anything. Any one of us can do this.

The discipline is not in making the promise but in keeping it. We have to be vigilant. We have to remember our promise not to suffer, sometimes every day, no matter what is going on around us. We may have to keep occupied with challenging activities to avoid getting caught up in thoughts or feelings. We cannot hang on to sentiment or symbols or behaviors that would shake us from our promise. We may have to watch how we speak so as not to elicit too much sympathy or pity from other people, which could upset us or shake us from our resolve not to suffer.

Know that the stand or promise not to suffer does not imply that we are heartless and cold, nor does it mean that we stop loving the people that we have lost. To promise not to suffer is just that. It is not a promise to give up loving or a promise to shut ourselves down. It is a promise that enables us to manage our feelings and reactions. Then we can be free to remember without pain, love without anguish, and go on without sorrow or regret.

When Laura declared herself complete with her deceased husband, she wanted to do something new, that she had never even considered doing before, and so she and a friend went backpacking in the Himalayas. After the trip, she told me that standing on the top of those mountains she was awed by the incredible beauty around her. It stunned her to realize she might never have seen all this beauty had she not been willing to leave her grief behind and stop suffering now.

There is enormous power available to us when we take a stand for ourselves and for our lives. Choosing not to suffer and living that commitment every day opens the door to new opportunities and new experiences. Choosing not to suffer is a profound statement of self-respect that generates vitality and joy instead of inertia, resignation, and despair. The commitment not to suffer powerfully enhances our lives. Unimaginable possibilities open up in declaring aloud, "I promise not to suffer anymore." Actually, great possibilities open up whenever we are willing to take a stand to alter our lives in any way.

In the next section, "How We Put Salt in Our Wounds," we will look at the behaviors that generate or extend our suffering, the pitfalls and the obstacles to living fulfilled. Having alluded to the certainty that we cause our own misery, in the next section we will examine specific ways we do that, beginning with our being right about suffering, and including dramatizing, personalizing, living in the past, self-tortures, and more. Again, let's read while remembering that each of us is human and knowing that each of us has three self-denying tendencies. Uncovering these common, automatic, and habitual behaviors can free us to live more successfully. The intention of this next part, as well as of the book as a whole, is to enhance our ability to choose to overcome or recover from the pains of life, to give up suffering, and to have the possibility of transforming painful experiences.

• II •

HOW WE PUT SALT IN OUR WOUNDS

• 6 •

BEING RIGHT ABOUT SUFFERING: WE WOULD RATHER BE RIGHT THAN HAPPY

It is not true that suffering ennobles the character;
happiness does that sometimes, but suffering,
for the most part, makes men petty and vindictive.
WILLIAM SOMERSET MAUGHAM, *THE MOON AND SIXPENCE*

Some people reading this book will find it very difficult to take the possibility of not suffering to heart. We do not think we can stop, so the idea of just stopping suffering upsets our whole belief system. This is one reason so much suffering persists in the world. We get stuck in our beliefs and our positions, and we will not stop. For instance, we may believe that life is hard or that pain persists forever, and no one can tell us otherwise. As a result, no matter how unhappy we are, we do not change or learn new ways to live.

To stop suffering may seem impossible. Our beliefs and our positionality—that is, our tendency to have a position or attitude about something and stick to it—are what most prevent us from ending our suffering, from healing and being complete. In hanging on to our beliefs and staying glued to our position, we make ourselves "right" for however we feel or act. Unpleasant as it may be to confront, most of us would rather be "right" than happy.

One woman I know literally went to bed for a year after her father died. She told me that withdrawing to her bed was her expression of grief. After her husband's death, another woman wore black for nearly fifty years, until her own death at eighty. One man spent twenty years in a constant state of bitterness and anger after his son's death. These people took positions in response to their grief that they held on to for years, positions that they thought were "right." To tell them that they did not have to suffer to this extent, that they had a choice, would have sounded absurd to them. I have had the experience several times of arguing with longtime attenders of bereavement groups who insist they will never get over their loss. My sense is that they will be "right" about that, no matter what other possibilities exist.

Telling any of these people, "You can stop suffering," might leave them feeling seriously misunderstood or even ridiculous for how they had been behaving. We will make whatever we do "right" to avoid being invalidated, to avoid feeling "wrong," which for most of us is a terrible feeling. Some of us will do anything to be right, anything to maintain our position, regardless of the degree of pain it causes us or other people. We mourn, criticize, label, hate, hold grudges, and withhold, all under the guise that we are right and another is wrong. At those times it matters more to be right than to be contented, vital, or loving.

Often we do not even know that we are entrenched in a position, for we get so used to our own ideas that they simply fit us. It may take a wake-up call from outside ourselves, a cue or reminder from someone else, for us to realize we are holding fast to a position. This book offers many "wake-up calls" and so may be uncomfortable reading at times.

It is important to realize that every one of us gets "stuck" in our own positions from time to time. That's human. We become entrenched in our own personal interpretations, our beliefs, or our attitudes about life. Problems arise when we cannot see our positions simply as a position, when we get "stuck" in thinking life is only the way we see it. Then we have no choice, no freedom, and we victimize ourselves unknowingly. Most destructive is to be "stuck" with the idea that we have to suffer, for that idea can cause us endless pain and ruin years of our lives.

DO YOU WANT TO STOP SUFFERING?

If, as we read this book, we see that we have been holding fast to some destructive ideas or positions, we have a choice of changing. Not all of us are going to be willing to stop suffering, so the first question to be asked is, "Do we want to stop hurting?" When I ask people that question, I am always surprised when they do not shout out an unequivocal "Yes!" Instead, people often look at me suspiciously, as if I am about to take away a favorite possession. We get very attached to our suffering, so this is no lightweight question.

The second part of that question is, "Do we want to stop suffering enough to be willing to give up being 'right'?" In other words, in giving up our suffering can we tolerate that we may feel invalidated or regretful? We may be sorry that we spent so much time feeling badly. Right away we can see that it may take courage to risk a different kind of discomfort, temporarily, if we are to give up suffering.

For several months in therapy with me, Ken struggled over letting go of his grief for his dead wife. Sometimes our discussions felt like power struggles as he held fast to his belief that he would never recover from this loss. One day I said to him, "Okay, Ken, you're right. You will never get over Ann's death." He immediately became angry that I would say such a thing, and then suddenly he laughed and said, "No, you're right. I am going to be just fine!" That is the stand that finally freed him from grief.

What can be significant in waking us up to let go of our self-righteousness is our honest desire to be finished with the past and to be satisfied with our lives today. Many of us truly do want to live fulfilled, but we do not know what it takes. Committing ourselves to living in the present and to having an ongoing completeness in our lives and in our relationships, instead of suffering, can afford us real freedom and satisfaction. That commitment alone would help release us from the everyday obstinacy to which most of us are prone. Instead of our usual self-righteousness, by competing to see who could change their position faster we would discover an amazing degree of harmony, intimacy, and contentment in our relationships.

The tendency to remain entrenched in the past is common to all of us, so common that we may not even notice it in ourselves and one another. However, that tendency is often how we maintain suffering for months or years beyond the original hurts. We will address "Living in the Past" next.

•7•

LIVING IN THE PAST

History's lessons are no more enlightening
than the wisdom of those who interpret them.
DAVID SCHOENBRUN

What makes it especially hard for us to recover from painful events is that we hang on to them, and we never forget. We keep our wounds open and alive, so that they eventually serve as walls between us and life. We tend to rerun a painful incident or our whole anguished story over and over, like a favorite movie, which constantly blurs out the present. Unknowingly we also use our past to determine the future, so that often there is no opportunity for something new to occur.

THE PAST IS OVER

Nothing we can do now can alter the past. All we can influence about the past is our interpretation of it. Yet we rehash events and feelings gone by as if they will somehow change. There would be no more to say about it except that most of us carry our history around with us as one of our most cherished possessions. We remember it, relieve it, and retell it. Worst of all, we torture ourselves over what we can no longer change or affect. The past is irrelevant except for what it has already taught us. Yet we often act as if the past matters more than today.

Once we live through a traumatic event, it is critical that we remember that it is over and past; it is usually a one-time-only occurrence in our lives. This is hard to do because we associate ourselves with our past all the time. History does not necessarily repeat itself, and yet sadly we await what we imagine to be the certainty of another traumatic incident occurring. If we lived through war, we may anticipate war. If we have been very poor, we may fear recurrent poverty. If we were abandoned, we may always be on guard for possible abandonments. If we have lost people, we may persistently dread loss. Since each of us lives through our own unique set of experiences, our feelings of fear or hurt are not triggered by the same events. We do not each worry about poverty or war or death, for we tend to fear what we have already known.

We all regularly use the past as a reference point. We keep looking backward to see how to operate our lives now, how we did it before, and how it turned out then. We use our history to either duplicate something that worked before or defend ourselves against something that did not work before. Sometimes we duplicate the past automatically because that is all we know to do. There is no aliveness and no chance for generating anything new in duplicating and defending. Since the past is but a series of memories that are likely to be distorted and narrow, what we remember is often inaccurate and fictionalized. Nonetheless, we attempt to orchestrate our lives out of this fiction all the time.

When our only reference is the past, we may not see or experience what is actually happening today. If we drove our automobiles using the rearview mirror as our only reference point, we would probably crash quickly. If we want to successfully drive a car, we must see more than what is behind us. This is true for directing our lives as well. The past should serve only as one of many reference points.

Most of us cling to our past, allowing it to indiscriminately run our future. We base our relationships now on what happened in our earlier relationships. We constantly associate and compare current people in our lives with past people, today's experiences with earlier experiences. Often without realizing it, we live today out of such past events as our fathers' leaving us or our mothers' dying or our being bullied or ignored. Even though these events occurred twenty or thirty or even fifty years ago, they are alive for us right now. Unfortunately, a lot of us are so nostalgic, so enmeshed in our stories from the past, that today does not have much of a chance.

Our persistent embracing, magnifying, and reliving of our past over and again is a major source of our suffering in life. Even though we are hurt by reminders from our history, that is what we usually talk about—our past losses, failures, and disappointments. Each telling reopens the pain, and yet the sad stories we rerun are often our favorite stories to tell.

Although nostalgia may seem enjoyable, sometimes there is a fine line between the pleasure and the torture in it. Many of us like to look at old photographs and tell anecdotes to recapture the sense of relationship, the experiences, the feelings, and especially the love that we felt in the past. Then we hurt. What seemed fun at first may evoke distress or sadness or grief over what we are missing now or what was missing then.

WE ARE ALWAYS INFLUENCED BY THE PAST

Although we may not be aware of it, we often base our whole lives on decisions resulting from just one uncomfortable past incident. We are deeply hurt by a buddy, so we decide not to be intimate anymore. We break a leg skiing, so we never ski again. A teacher or relative inadvertently embarrasses us in front of other people, so we decide never to speak in public again. We experience poverty, so all the rest of our lives is about amassing things to make up for it. Our parents take away our dog, so as an adult we become a dog breeder. We are so upset or helpless in dealing with an irrational or erratic parent that we eventually become a counselor or psychiatrist. Our lives are literally filled with examples like these, illustrating how much we live today based on the past, whether we recognize it or not.

What is particularly dramatic is that one single upsetting incident can influence a person for the rest of his or her life. One shout, one error, one fall, one rejection can be the basis from which we build or inhibit all future relationships. As a therapist, I often hear stories about how lives were "ruined" by a cruel, demanding teacher or parent, how one humiliating incident altered life forever, how an accident years ago plagues us today, how the loss of a childhood love caused us never to love again. We seem more than willing to stop our vitality or give up on life because of one painful moment or event.

Remember, we create the suffering in our lives after upsetting events occur. It is how we use painful events, what we do with them later, that hurts us. Jo's mother died of cancer and, not surprisingly, Jo's major fear in every one of her subsequent relationships was that she would be abandoned—again. As a result many different kinds of behaviors in people, like lateness, wanting time alone, and changing plans, all looked to Jo like abandonment. Jo lives in a self-fulfilling prophesy. By unknowingly immortalizing her past trauma, she herself keeps recreating her dreaded sense of abandonment. Though she may not think so, Jo is a victim of herself, of her own thoughts and beliefs, and not a victim of other people's insensitivity or cruelty.

We can easily be victims of our history. Many of us are dominated by our previous experiences without realizing it. Traumatic events linger. Even when we cannot remember it, an earlier hurt, shock, or unusual event can provoke feelings today. Part of why these events linger and are not resolved is that we may have had no way to express and release our reactions to upsetting incidents when they occurred.

Incomplete reactions from childhood are natural. We all bring with us to adulthood stored up past reactions that we could not communicate. Psychotherapy can help us detach today's attitudes and feelings from past events. We can also do that for ourselves now, if we pay attention to our reactions. Whenever we overreact today, we can attempt to remember the source by asking ourselves: What does this remind me of? Even if we do not remember, we can feel freer today just knowing that this reaction is probably, in part, a throwback to the past.

We can separate ourselves from our past when we are willing to take charge of our lives and live in the present. Only when we distinguish for ourselves that we have a history, and that we are not our history, is it possible for us to be fully alive now without indulging in the allure of our past. Of course, reminders will evoke the past sometimes, for some of our memories do last forever. However, we can shortcut our reactions by being aware that we have a choice: to live our experiences as they occur today, or to persist in reacting to and from some other earlier time.

SHIFTING HOW WE REGARD OUR PAST

Here is where our imagination can serve as a powerful tool, for we can use it to picture ourselves any way we wish to be.

Why not then remember the past as happy? Most of us seem to remember more of the unpleasant aspects than the happier times gone by. What we remember is likely to be fiction anyway. Knowing this, we might consider that it is never too late to have a happy childhood, which we can do by consciously remembering and reminding ourselves of happy days past. We may want to repeat these imaginings over and over to combat our negativity and to make them more real.

If we cannot remember good times, we can make them up or rewrite our story by changing how we remember past times. Instead of remembering high school as a time of low self-esteem and loneliness, we could picture ourselves as feeling more confident and having good companions. Instead of thinking of ourselves as the least loved of our siblings, we might create ourselves as our parents' most beloved child. In so doing, we may even discover that that was closer to the truth. Writing our lives as a fairy tale or a short story is another way to purposely evoke earlier happy days.

We can consciously elect to create today what we missed in the past. We can find the missing love, nourishment, companionship, fun, challenge, risk, respect, and the like in generating new relationships and new experiences to satisfy ourselves now. We do not have to persist in living with "missing pieces" from the past, for we can take the responsibility to make up for what we missed or lost. We have to be the ones to fill in the gaps in our lives, and in so doing we are designers, not victims any longer.

WE CAN STOP LIVING AS OUR HISTORY

All of us act now out of the past. We do things because we did them before. Our preferences and tastes come out of the past. For example, we often eat from memory. If we stop and notice, we will see that we eat what we remember that we like. We may not taste today's food at all. A good experiment would be to taste a variety of foods today, newly, as if we never tasted them before. We might discover new or different tastes and more pleasure in eating. This kind of experimenting can be useful in other areas as well. We can look at our tastes, interests, and choices of people, activities, and places to begin to experience who we are right now, freshly or newly, instead of relying on our past experiences to direct today. We can be much more alive to today by experiencing the present instead of dwelling in the past.

When we are willing to be responsive to and responsible for our lives, we can have our history without being immersed in it or dominated by it. The greatest gift we can give ourselves is to be complete and finished with all that has occurred before. Chapter 23, "Completing Our Experiences," will be particularly valuable to this end. The most freeing and empowering stand we can take in regard to our history is to admit and live from the truth that the past is over.

•8•

LIVING IN THE FUTURE

It isn't the experience of today that drives men mad.
It is the remorse for something that happened yesterday,
and the dread of what tomorrow may disclose.
ROBERT JONES BURDETTE, *THE GOLDEN DAY*

Living in the future is just as destructive as living in the past. Just as we get tripped up by our history, we also add to our suffering by what in Gestalt therapy is called "futurizing." We project this moment, this behavior, this trauma, this conflict into the future, and we anticipate endless and lasting pain or misery for ourselves. Futurizing is one way we cope with the uncomfortable reality that our future is an unknown, but it results in self-torture.

OUR FUTURE IS UNKNOWN

Most of us do a great deal of worrying or daydreaming about or planning for the future. We want to be prepared. We anticipate how we will cope with an imagined job loss or financial failure or the threat of losing someone we love. We miss enjoying, and sometimes we even wreck, our relationships because we are so afraid of losing them. We try to prepare for events the reality of which we cannot even imagine. I spent years trying to be ready for the deaths of my parents only to discover that the reality was different from and actually easier than any of my imaginings.

We are not expert forecasters of our lives, and yet we live as if we have powerful predictive powers. Notice how many things we projected in to the future that never came to pass— all the losses we anticipated or the frightening scenarios we created regarding lack of money or lack of love. How often we anticipated that if we were honest with someone the relationship would be in jeopardy. Yet this kind of honesty generally brings us closer together, not farther apart. Instead of knowing the future, usually we are surprised by how our lives turn out, surprised by the turns, curves, and events that occur on our road of life.

EXAMINING THE FUTURE

The following exercise can demonstrate how poorly we forecast our future. Let's stop and look at our lives exactly as they are now, scanning all their aspects: relationships with family and friends, work, home, life-style, and activities. Then let's ask ourselves, "Is this where I expected to be today?" or "Five years ago (or ten or twenty years ago), is this what I expected to have or be or do now?" Chances are that how life has turned out so far is unexpected and filled with people, things, and events that we could never have anticipated in advance.

I am awed reflecting on the changes in my own life since writing this book. Alone earlier, I suspected I might always live alone writing books. We always think now will persist into the future. Instead, I married the kind of man I never before dreamed existed. This is another example of how we do not know what the future holds for us.

Another way to see our relationships with the past and future is to remember ourselves at some young age—seven or ten or fourteen. Remember who we were and what we wanted in life then. For a moment let's be ten with a ten-year-old's dreams. At ten, I wanted to live with a husband on some vast estate with lots of servants and raise dogs—a laughable idea to me now. That was a ten-year-old's dream of being grown-up, which would bore me today. At ten, none of us could predict who we are now.

Our lives today undoubtedly include many people and experiences that we would never have known to predict or desire earlier. We have jobs, friends, a spouse, children, and homes that are nothing like what we imagined ahead of time. Life is unpredictable, so trying to determine it mentally in advance is a waste of time. Again, we are bound to be unhappy when we allow ourselves to be distracted by the past or the future.

• 9 •

ROMANTICIZING

*I never cease being dumbfounded by
the unbelievable things people believe.*

LEO ROSTEN

We are a society of romantics. We tend to fight reality
instead of grasping it and accepting it, which makes
dealing with the hurts of life all the more difficult. Our ongoing romanticizing of life is a pitfall that trips us up over and over
again. It is one of the ways we victimize ourselves, and it is a
major source of suffering.

Most of us would say we are realists. We'd say, "I know how
it is in life" or "I call a spade a spade." We are mostly unaware
of how romantic we are about life. Yet we can see our lack of
realism in how we deal with disappointments and tragedies.
We invariably talk about how something should not or could
not have happened instead of allowing or including what has
occurred.

We speak with a lot of romantic expressions. We can hear
our romanticizing of tragic or upsetting events when we say, "I
wish," "I hope," "Maybe it will change," "Maybe it isn't true," "It
could not have happened," "It would have been different if," or

"If only." The most powerful of these are our hoping "if only"s and clinging to sentiment.

HOPE

We try to make real life go away with hope. While circumstances are crashing in around us, we hope. We hope that maybe it was a mistake or perhaps things will change or get better. When our relationships are in trouble, we hope they will improve. When we hear bad news, we hope it isn't true. When tragedy strikes, we hope it will go away. When someone leaves us we think, with no basis in reality, that just maybe he or she will come back. For example, even after his divorce was finalized and his former wife had moved to another city, my client Joe imagined she would come back to him. He hurt anew each day she did not return. It took him many months to face that he was living in a fairy tale, in hope instead of in real life.

Instead of acting to improve our lives, we live hoping and waiting for life to turn out as we would like it to be. We live in hope while relationships are not working or funds are limited or terrible crises impend. Hope is usually just fantasy and is the stance of a passive victim. There is no power in hope, no action and no healing ourselves with hope, and yet many of us cling to it like a life raft.

"IF ONLY"S

We universally focus our attention on what we are missing rather than on what we have, the way we wish life to be instead of the way it is. We discount reality by envisioning that it could be otherwise. When confronted with pain, we attempt to avoid or rewrite or fix the moment by saying, "If only it were different."

We use "If only"s in an attempt to make the present more bearable, particularly after tragedies, deaths, and crises occur. We say things like, "If only I knew ahead of time," "If only he hadn't gone," or "If only I was driving instead." When someone dies, we imagine rewriting the facts to resurrect the dead person. Then we say things like, "If only I had taken him to the doctor sooner," or worse, "If only it had been me, not him." We torture ourselves this way, imagining that we can resurrect or recreate what we have lost.

We try to empower ourselves with "if only"s especially when we feel most powerless. We may get some kind of solace from our momentary sense of control or power in attempting to rewrite our lives, and yet employing "if only"s in the face of a crisis ultimately makes confronting reality all the more difficult. When we avoid the true facts, it takes us longer to accept and finish with them. "If only"s delay our healing time and keep us locked in unproductive imaginings.

Even though "if only"s do not help us, it may seem hard to stop these ideas. We can stop this and other unproductive ways of thinking by staying alert to our indulging in this kind of fantasy, by not making these thoughts so significant, and by consciously distracting ourselves from our thoughts. The most important tool in dissuading us from "if only"s is our willingness to allow our reality to be as it is instead of playing games in our minds to try to change it.

SENTIMENT

We also exaggerate our pain when we romanticize after tragedies and losses by clinging to any reminders of the one we lost. We tend to cling to photographs, letters, momentos, and memories. We listen intently to sad songs that express or even glorify our pain. We are so caught up in our sentiments that we then find it difficult to accept the reality of our loss and harder still to let go and go on anew.

We enshrine our dead loved one's belongings, or read old letters over and over, or moon over photographs instead of going out into life today. This is overly sentimentalizing, and it does not help at all. It's like adding salt to a wound. In my work with people in grief, it has become evident that extensive sentimentality, that grasping too tightly the reminders of our loss, delays our healing. In being attached to sentiment, memories, or mementos, we are living in the past and reliving our loss over and over. As a result, we have no freedom to expand, to heal, and to go on with our lives. This does not mean that we should destroy all the photographs, letters, and mementos from the past. It means that if we want to recover quickly we should look at them sparingly, not all the time. Again, living now, not living with symbols from the past, is the healthiest choice we can make.

EVERYDAY ROMANTICIZING

Our lack of realism is not just in the face of tragedy, but is an everyday affair. Frequently there is a discrepancy between how we envision life to be and how life actually is. Because of our romantic views, real life is often disappointing and sometimes very distressing. Much of our suffering over our lives results from our longing for life to be ideal instead of real, wishing we were superhuman, without human problems, needs, or feelings.

Real life is full of the unexpected, so it can be frustrating, upsetting, boring, and disheartening. Worst of all, life can present sudden, unforeseen turns of fate like accidents and illnesses, changes and losses. Since we need to be able to cope with all that life embodies, our romanticizing sabotages us.

Because we do not admit that life hurts and can thwart us, we are unprepared to face tragedy, loss, and disappointment. We tend to avoid or resist "real" life when it confronts us head-on because it does not fit into our picture of how life is supposed to be. As a result, we do not learn to develop our abilities to handle life's confrontations until we are forced to do so. Usually whatever we learn about mastering life comes by chance or accident, the result of trial and error.

Being human is no easy task. Each of us needs to be able to deal with real-life experiences as they occur and then recover. We can do so when we let life be as it is instead of fighting it. We would do best taking on the challenge that life is instead of trying to hide from it through illusion and fantasy. We would be stronger if we avoided living out of hope, sentiment, or fantasy. For, more than anything else, accepting life as an opportunity is a major pathway out of suffering.

• 10 •

SEARCHING FOR MEANING

It was previously a question of finding out whether or not life had to have a meaning to be lived. It now becomes clear, on the contrary, that it will be lived all the better if it has no meaning.

ALBERT CAMUS

E ven though there is no meaning built into life, each of us adds meaning to everything, to everyday events, to our own and other people's behaviors, feelings, and attitudes, as well as to illnesses, tragedies, and other unexpected events. We do not allow our experiences just to be whatever they are; we make them *mean* something. We imagine that finding some kind of reason or answer will give us solace, enhance our lives, and resolve our difficulties. Unfortunately, this search for meaning or reasons or answers backfires, for we end up with little relief or resolution. We may or may not get insight into our circumstances, but we get no help in dealing with the present reality.

SEEKING MEANING BY ASKING, "WHY?"

Asking "Why?" is the most obvious way we seek meaning. In the midst of tragic or disturbing experiences we invariably stop and question: "Why Me? Why is this happening now?

What is the meaning of this?" We assume that "why" is a useful question and that there is an answer that will somehow assist or relieve us. We imagine that once we find an answer, we will be released from our feelings of distress.

This almost never works. Answers may give us moments of awareness or insight, but no relief. Instead we have information, an interpretation that we have made up, information that may actually intensify our anguish. When people suffer a loss, they invariably ask why the person died. The answer they fabricate may make them feel worse. To imagine the person died because they couldn't bear to be married anymore or because of a crisis at work or because their children didn't do enough for them puts unjustified blame on a spouse or children or a boss and leaves everyone feeling upset and powerless to cope with the loss.

Asking "Why?" is a way to assign blame, as if we will resolve anything or generate any relief by pinpointing who or what is to blame. We ask, "Why am I sick? Why did the accident occur? Why did he leave? Why did she say that?" If we actually discover or know why, does that really help or change anything? Without a doubt this is one way we torture ourselves in dealing with crises or problems. For this reason I call "why"s "the killer questions," for they kill our aliveness and our resourcefulness and leave us frustrated, powerless, and unresolved.

The meanings we add often hurt us rather than support us. Notice how we commonly torment ourselves after a relationship ends. We invent reasons for the ending that undermine us, such as not having been lovable enough or good enough or loving enough, or reasons that invalidate the other person, such as that they were too immature or too inflexible or too needy. Then, must we confront not only this loss but also our demeaning ideas about inadequacies in our ability to choose or to be loved.

Questioning upsetting events tends to intensify our distress since no explanation really suffices. We may justify why we were singled out to suffer, but instead of being relieved, we feel worse. Asking "why?" as we do, we seek out fruitless answers, instead of confronting the present moment squarely in order to resolve it. When we face and experience life head-on, we are free to fully react and then to let it go right then and there. Our pain is over. Not so when we ask "Why?"

The only accurate answer to all "why" questions is "because," period. Anything we add then, any other explanation, generates fiction and may cause us more trouble than the event we are questioning. Actually, if we look we will see that knowing an answer does not alter the circumstances in question.

THE POWER OF NOT ADDING MEANING

Therefore, speaking just the facts with nothing added can be a powerful tool in our coping more easily with our circumstances. Whatever happened simply happened. Free of added meaning, events can be dealt with, managed, and released without the usual intensity, distress, and drama that our interpretations usually create. We could cope more ably with whatever our circumstances—illness, death, or tragedy—if we did not waste our time worrying about why these events occurred. We would probably heal more quickly, too.

A great secret of mastering life is to give up adding meaning to all the occurrences in our lives. To achieve that we would have to relinquish our right to interpret every incident and to then believe our own interpretations. We might begin experimenting now with not adding anything extra to our reactions or experiences. When something upsetting happens, we can practice stating just the facts and speaking simply and specifically about our feeling with no elaboration: I hurt because I hurt. I am angry because I am angry. I fell because I fell. He died because he died. The accident happened because it happened.

I am convinced that tough circumstances are easier to take and quicker to resolve when we simply deal with the actuality, the event or experience itself, adding nothing extra. We can live through illness, accident, loss, even catastrophe, coping all the more easily, when we hold them to be just what has happened, giving them no additional meaning or interpretation.

MAKING LIFE MEANINGFUL: HAVING A PURPOSE

There is a paradox about adding meaning to life. We can see the destructiveness of the meanings and interpretations we add to life's events. On the other hand, by adding a sense of purpose to our lives we create a sense of meaning that enhances our lives. Having a purpose for living can help us find the courage to go on, no matter what life events or obstacles we confront. How we make our lives meaningful or worthwhile with purpose is elaborated in chapter 27, "Recovering by Structuring Our Lives with Purpose."

Clearly, then, it is the kind of meaning that we add to life that can impede or enhance our experience, and unfortunately most of the meanings we add interfere with our satisfaction and generate suffering. To further demonstrate this point, another destructive kind of added meaning, "Personalizing," is addressed in the next chapter.

• 11 •

PERSONALIZING

Change your thoughts and you change your world.
NORMAN VINCENT PEALE

Another common trouble-making reaction is personalizing, which is when we interpret and misinterpret everything that occurs in terms of its impact on us. It hurts us when we imagine other people are "doing it to us" because they themselves are upset, distracted, angry, or reacting in some way. Our personalizing is demonstrated whenever we think life's events or other's actions are about us or at us or to us. Personalizing the impersonal events of life is guaranteed to intensify our suffering, especially when we decide that we were singled out to experience tragedies or disappointments. Asking "Why me?" when upsetting things happen is a particularly virulent form of personalizing.

We assign blame or responsibility for circumstances or events, for at the root of personalizing is our search for causation or meaning. Personalizing serves to single us out as special and to separate us as wronged or misunderstood. A common form of this is when we say something like, "It rained, so I must not have been meant to take the trip." The rain was not meant especially for us. There is no relationship between the rain and the trip, but we put the two into a causative relationship.

Mishearing or misinterpreting is another aspect of personalizing. There are times when we dismiss reality and write it our own way. Yet, most of us are not aware of the extent to which we personalize. Some of us only personalize when we are feeling low or vulnerable, while others of us automatically personalize all of our experiences and interactions with each other all the time. An extreme example is my friend Carrie, who always asks, "Why did you say that?" for she imagines that whatever people talk about is directed personally at her. If you talk about older women to Carrie, she thinks that you mean she is old—even though she is thirty. Another example of personalizing was Flo, who blamed her husband, Jack, for losing his excess weight to hurt her. She was sure he lost weight to make himself unattractive to her, while Jack's weight loss enhanced his own self-esteem.

We personalize events that are only tangentially related to us, such as when we say the weather or the car dealer or the supermarket all "did it to us." We personalize the weather by acting as if the rain were attacking us individually. We think the car dealer selected us alone as a "sucker" or that the supermarket is purposely out of the products we wanted. We personalize upsetting occurrences as if we were singled out to have a flat tire or miss our bus or have our basement flooded or have our purse stolen. This kind of personalizing is a subtle source of a lot of our suffering in life. Events can be tough to manage, but personalizing makes them harder still.

WHY ME? PITY AND SELF-PITY

One of the most treacherous and tormenting questions we ask ourselves in the face of upsetting circumstances is "Why me?"

Asking "Why me?" sets up a self-pitying cycle, implying how we ordinarily feel singled out to suffer. This is the height of personalizing. Pity and self-pity debilitate and deplete us and deprive us of confidence, and we are invariably left with a sense of ourselves as powerless victims of fate rather than masters of life.

In our culture self-pity seems to be a natural, even fundamental, part of our relationship to upsetting events. We feel sorry for ourselves when we hurt in any way, as if hurt is inhuman and unnatural. How often we console each other with words like, "You poor thing," or "How awful for you." We see ourselves and one another as victims. When others feel sorry for us, it validates and confirms that we are really suffering, that we are special, or that we are worse off than other people. In actuality, our own and other people's pity keep us "stuck" and unable to come to terms with our pain.

The question "Why me?" reflects our tendency to compare ourselves and our lives with those of other people, when our lives are never comparable. Each of us is actually on our own path, having our own experiences. Comparisons are another way we torture ourselves with the idea that life could be other than how it is.

Self-pity is a reaction over which we can have a choice, for we can choose not to pity ourselves or others. More empowering than asking "Why me?" would be to ask ourselves, "Why shouldn't life challenge me just as it challenges anyone else? Or even more than anyone else?" Challenge is vital to our growth and development. Unchallenged, we would sit around in life, immobile, bored, constricted, and lifeless. Therefore, a more important question for us to consider is "Why not me?"

OTHER FORMS OF PERSONALIZING

We see our experiences in terms of rewards and punishments, another way we add meaning and personalize. We see hardships, losses, and illnesses as punishments, and falling in love or having money or success as rewards. The bad news about life is that there are no rewards, and the good news is that there are no punishments. We make all of that up through our own interpretations, and this becomes evident when we see that a reward for one of us might be a punishment to another.

We personalize circumstances and the actions of others. If someone forgets to return a telephone call, we take it as a rejection. If our spouse or our child is crabby because of a bad day at work or school, we interpret their behavior as being hurtful to us. If our child fails or behaves badly, we assume it is our fault. If a loved one dies, we feel singled out to suffer loss or, even more extreme, we imagine they did it to affect us or hurt us. Our lives are loaded with examples just like these of which we are usually unaware.

We personalize what other people say, and then we react out of what we think we hear. If someone says they are upset, we imagine they are upset with us. If an intimate expresses feelings, we turn that into some error we have committed rather than hearing about them. We often cannot hear each other because we are so focused on ourselves. I contend that most of us are poor listeners, even those of us like lawyers, physicians, educators, and psychotherapists who are trained to listen to others. We are often too preoccupied with ourselves and our own inner dialogue to really hear what another is saying and meaning.

When we personalize we add ourselves into our experiences, particularly in upsetting or tough circumstances. This is one way we make ourselves important or special, or at least establish our own unique mark or identity on our experiences. Unfortunately, when we assume that we were specially singled out, we make the incidents or accidents of life personal events and all the more distressing or painful.

Personalizing diminishes our power and compounds our pain. When we blame ourselves for circumstances that are out of our control, we make ourselves out to be victims. Singled out, we are victims, and life is always harder from the vantage point of a victim. We are equally off balance when we imagine someone else "made us" angry or caused our feelings. Assigning responsibility outside of ourselves limits our power to confront our circumstances. We can see that personalizing is harmful, serving only to ascribe meaning, useless meaning.

THE POSSIBILITY OF NOT PERSONALIZING

Maybe we don't have to function this way. Compare ourselves with our pets. I stepped on my Newfoundland dog's toe one day, and she yelped. That was the beginning and the end of the incident for her. If someone hurts our feelings or disappoints us, we don't just yelp. We immediately add weight to the moment by personalizing it, saying or thinking "How could you!" or "Why did you do that?" or "You did that on purpose!" Then we keep reexamining ourselves to see if we are damaged. We dramatize the incident by telling others about it, sometimes many times over. We don't simply yelp and then let go of pain. If we did, this would be the surest means to be complete with our experiences and not to suffer.

We can choose whether or not to personalize distressing events, even though we are usually unaware of having any choice over this behavior. It can be truly life-transforming to choose whether or not to see any of life's circumstances as something being done especially to us. Notice the distinction between "my husband is angry right now" and "my husband must be angry at me." There is such a big difference between saying "my mother died" and "I felt abandoned by my mother when she died." The first sentence in each pair expresses the fact or event. The second is what we might add to it, implying what was done to us. Imagine how differently these two ways of speaking could affect how we experience our mothers' deaths, for example, or how differently we would experience anything in life if we were clear it was not about us or at us.

We can overcome personalizing by being alert for it in our daily lives. We can listen for who or how we blame when an upsetting event occurs. We can notice how often we or other people ask, "What did I do to cause this?" We will begin to see the absurdity in how we assign blame for rain or someone else's anger or our flooded basement. We can learn to distinguish when we are imagining something is being done to us or is about us.

Noticing what we react to time and again is another useful means of gaining power over our reactions. We can be in charge once we notice that "I always seem to get angry when I'm ignored" or "when I'm criticized" or "when I have to wait." We can see that "I feel defensive when I am corrected" or "when I am called upon unexpectedly" or "when people make suggestions to me." Another aspect of looking at ourselves is to see that "whenever somebody yells [or cries or is late or changes their mind] I feel hurt." We tend to react to the same kind of things all the time. Once I saw that I always reacted with anger or defensiveness to being told what to do or to being criticized,

I could then prevent myself from falling into the same traps over and over. Now I actually relish other people's criticisms or advice as contributions to me.

Ownership always begins with the word "I" and follows from an objective observation of ourselves and how we behave or react. Instead of being like automatons that react to the same events again and again, it is exciting to watch ourselves so as to gain power over our reactions and our lives. It would be very valuable for us to stop and notice whatever we react to time and again, so that we can begin to manage that behavior more successfully for ourselves.

If we could be aware enough of ourselves to do so, one important way of not personalizing in our relationships is to listen objectively to how the other person experiences life, apart from us, instead of insinuating ourselves into what they say. The best metaphor is that we are all players on the same baseball team, and yet the game looks different from each position or perspective, different to the catcher than to the outfielder or the pitcher. If we would simply listen to how each of us sees the "game," we could hear each other, and we could feel free to report the "game" from our perspective as well. This way we could have a powerful means of communicating. Communicating is not as difficult or scary or hurtful when we do not personalize what other people say.

Lastly, being clear about our responsibility frees us from personalizing. As has been noted earlier, responsibility is taking charge of how we respond or how we handle our reactions to the events that occur. We can be responsible for our own personal responses, not for the event itself. Our responsibility involves living through and owning our feelings as they occur rather than seeing ourselves as victims of our emotions. Our ownership of our reactions can powerfully alter our experience of our circumstances. When we know that we always are upset by rain or other people's anger, we are no longer thrown off by these events. When we see our impatience in waiting or our fear of criticism or our dislike for being told what to do, we are no longer victims who think people are purposely out to get us. When we see that we were not singled out for a car accident or illness, we have more power to cope and recover.

Looking at the whole concept of personalizing is provocative and useful. Each of us might stop and take some time now to look at the ways he or she personalizes events or communications with other people. Several people did just that after reading the working manuscript of this book. One reader, whom I will call Lilly, noticed a dramatic shift in how she viewed her mother's coldness to her. For the first time she saw that her mother was in fact cold to everyone, a woman who allowed very little intimacy into her life, and that Lilly was not singled out to be treated this way. After having this insight, Lilly noticed that she was more relaxed in all her relationships with people—customers on her job as well as friends. She saw that she was no longer ruled by the idea that she was somehow unlovable because her mother had been cold to her. She is more trusting now, and she's having more fun with people than she ever did before.

Examining whatever it is that we personalize and taking responsibility for it can afford us a new freedom in life as well. I recommend that we each take time now to look at our own personalizing as a possible source of our own suffering in life before going on the next chapter, "Dramatizing."

• 12 •

DRAMATIZING

All the world's a stage, And all the men and women merely players.

SHAKESPEARE, *AS YOU LIKE IT*

L
ike personalizing, we are also prone, often unknowingly, to
dramatizing or embellishing our experiences. Although dramatizing may seem to make our lives more interesting or exciting, this hurts us. We increase our suffering by intensifying our
emotions, magnifying our upsets, and adding weight to our reactions and experiences. Our elaborations entrench us in our story
and can even extend the time it take us to recover.

Dramatizing is so common in our society that most everyone does it without noticing it. We dramatize in three ways—
by the words we use to describe everything in our lives, by
embellishing the facts, and by repeating the same incidents over
and over in creative and dramatic stories. We joke that "my life
is a soap opera," and unfortunately we are telling the truth.

THE WORDS WE USE

Our usage of words is the most common way we dramatize. We
typically overstate our experiences by the adjectives we add in

portraying them, as when we describe our lives with words like "horrible," "terrible," "worst," and "catastrophic." Even commonly used words like "very" or "most" have a dramatic quality in that they add something to the facts. We see the pervasiveness of this kind of exaggeration in our everyday news stories, as well as in most of our conversations with one another.

EMBELLISHING THE FACTS

In addition to the specific words we use, we may be unaware that we also dramatize by adding details to the facts. We can quickly turn an upsetting event into a tragedy by embellishing our feelings and elaborating on the story of our suffering. We do not simply and directly state, "I am hurt" or disappointed or angry or whatever. We add our opinions, outrage, and self-righteous thoughts to our feelings, expanding and intensifying our discomfort. Then we make up a story elaborating on and often justifying why we are hurt or disappointed, and we tell a lot of people. This is how we generate upsetting dramas and turn our lives into unmanageable soap operas. This is one of the ways we make our intimate relationships a source of suffering: We dramatize our disagreements and differences, exaggerating our problems out of all proportion, so that it makes it very hard to come to any resolution with one another.

How we speak about our lives deeply affects how we experience them. Usually we speak to one another out of our soap operas, elaborating on our experiences rather than stating the facts. To say, "I was in an automobile accident and injured my knee" is so different than what we would ordinarily say: "I was in a terrible car crash and nearly died." To say, "Ron and I are having difficulty communicating" or "we disagreed" is so different from elaborating on the argument so as to make the other person look like a jerk or from exaggerating the content.

REPEATING AND SOLIDIFYING OUR STORY

Not only do we exaggerate and expand upon the truth but we also tell our story over and over. A hairdresser I knew told every customer all day long whatever story she was working on at the moment. She would keep repeating the details about her dealings with her difficult mother or a fight she had with her husband or the bad behavior of her child. Dramatizing this way may have looked to her as a means of relief, but actually added weight to her problems and kept all of her relationships in turmoil and unresolved—not to mention how trying it was to be her audience and listen to her stories, which all were so negative and hopeless.

When we are grieving or very upset, we are apt to elaborate on or keep repeating the story of what happened. We often need to express ourselves to other people to relieve or release some of the pain—at first. This is a common and healthy reaction to a shocking event, initially. But if we continue speaking this way much too long, we extend our grief or pain. We could recover ourselves more quickly if after a few weeks we stopped talking about our pain as a story. That way we could be present to today and not have our grief be so preoccupying and persistent.

WE LIVE OUR LIVES AS CONTINUING DRAMAS

Many of us live in ongoing dramas, stories from the past rather than being present to life as a new experience from moment to moment. This is so common that we may not notice how often people glorify their college days or war stories or adolescent experiences years later. I remember a man of forty-two who told me the story of how he hated his mother as if he were still an outraged ten-year-old, and I remember the woman who vividly described her life with her husband, who died twenty years ago, as if he were with her today. How many parents talk about their children as they were years ago and seem to ignore who their offspring are now? We may live in yesterday's stories, day after day, or even tell the same story for years after an incident. Our lives become a series of stories *about* ourselves and our experiences instead of moments we live in or pass through or finish as they occur. There is no vitality, no joy, and no possibility for growth in living in stories of the past.

The benefits of dramatizing: Nonetheless, dramatizing runs rampant in our world since most of us relate to and engage one another by dramatizing. The benefit is that we indirectly get other people's attention, agreement, sympathy, assistance, or love. Our dramatizing may also seem to make our lives more exciting or interesting. This may be the only way we know to interact with other people, and it often seems we get more attention for the stories of our troubles than for those of our accomplishments and victories.

The detriments of dramatizing: Yet the subtle damage we do to ourselves in viewing our lives as dramas that happen to us is that we enlist one another in the widely held belief that we are all innocent victims of fate. As innocent bystanders in our lives, we can be both helpless and blameless. We are free of responsibility. Most of us avoid owning distressing occurrences because we tend to confuse responsibility or ownership with blame. We loathe and fear the idea that we caused a tragic event or deserved it as a punishment or retribution. However, the idea of retribution is simply another way we personalize or dramatize life events, another meaning we ourselves add.

Coping without dramatizing: After both my parents died, a friend asked me if I "felt like an orphan now." I saw both the drama she was offering me and how upsetting it might be to see myself that way. I chose not to feel sorry for myself that my parents' lives had come to their natural ends. Adding nothing extra for myself with which to contend, I completed my grief more quickly. I consciously chose not to dramatize my experience, which is a choice we all can make, once we are aware of it.

Not only are upsetting events easier for us when we do not dramatize them, but we also may have an easier time with other people. By not embellishing our experiences, we then do not provoke unwanted responses from others. When we are authentic and stick to the facts, other people usually do not leap to rescue us or pity us or avoid us. Then there is the possibility for real sharing and intimacy. Other people's responses to our tragedies, depending on what they are, can make it easier or harder for us to cope. Many of us have felt abandoned when we were suffering because others couldn't tolerate our tears or other emotions. It may be that if we were less dramatic others would be more available to us and more understanding. Certainly other people will not be as dramatic or as overly helpful and annoying if we don't provoke them with our own dramas.

Speaking just the straight facts—"I had an accident," "I broke my leg," "My father died," "My husband and I are separated"—reminds us that our experiences in themselves do not innately have to be cause for suffering. Owning our experiences and speaking simply and authentically can enable us to cope with life with more power, more courage, and more ease. I contend that we can overcome upsetting experiences much more easily when we do not dramatize them. We can begin today to experiment with not adding drama to our lives and see what a difference that change in our behavior makes. We will look next at other ways we add salt to our wounds, with behaviors that act as "self-tortures."

• 13 •

TORTURING OURSELVES

We have met the enemy and they are us.

POGO

We are being our own worst enemy whenever we indulge in what Fritz Perls, the originator of Gestalt therapy, called "self-tortures." Coping by indulging in destructive thinking processes, such as obsessive thinking, complaining, worry, regret, and guilt, can consume us and make us feel powerless to control our lives. I have noticed with many clients that once we see that our behaviors are "self-tortures" they lose their appeal and their power over our lives.

Self-torturing behaviors are usually so automatic that we may not have known until now that they deplete our energy and impede our handling of our lives. Therefore, the concept of "self-torture" itself may be startling or upsetting. Up to now, we may have felt at home with feelings of worry, guilt, or regret, or we may not have even noticed that we complain. The purpose in uncovering these behaviors is to free us to choose, if we wish, to let them go and to find more satisfying ways of dealing with life.

The Merriam-Webster Dictionary defines torture as "the act or process of inflicting severe pain, esp. as a punishment . . .

anguish of body or mind; agony. . . ." Self-torture then involves behaving in such a way that we inflict pain, anguish, or agony on ourselves, intending to punish ourselves or to coerce ourselves to act in some particular way. Although we torture ourselves inadvertently, the result is that often the least safe place for us to be is alone with ourselves. This will become more evident as we look at specific self-tortures like obsessive thinking, worry, and regret.

OBSESSIVE THINKING

What we call "thinking things out" is often simply a process by which our ideas run in circles. Our minds repeat ideas over and over, sometimes operating like machines that get stuck in one gear too long. This repetitive kind of thinking is obsessive thinking. We all do it. We can obsess about almost anything—any experience, reaction, feeling, thought, or memory. The more turmoil or stress we are experiencing, the more apt we are to obsess. Whenever something upsetting occurs or we have a difficult problem to solve, our minds suddenly fill with thoughts. Then we think about our problem constantly, as if we have no control over our thoughts.

Without our being aware of it, our repetitive thoughts may adversely affect our lives, for obsessive thinking keeps us awake at night and distracted during the day. We become victims of our own thought processes, imprisoned by our style of thinking. Instead of coming to a valuable conclusion or resolution, we simply end up thinking in circles, torturing ourselves. We allow ourselves to obsess because we believe that we have no control over how we think or that we need to "think things through" this way. We do not. We may have to learn to distract ourselves and to develop more effective means of problem solving.

Managing obsessive thinking by distracting ourselves: Although we may not believe it until we try it, it is possible to stop obsessive thinking and thus be free from a great deal of mental anguish. The way to reach resolution and peace of mind is to not give weight to our thoughts, to not listen to ourselves, to distract ourselves from thinking. We can distract ourselves by doing some other involving activity—a sport, reading, remembering and reliving something more satisfying, or challenging our minds with some other even more difficult problem, like thinking about the theory of relativity. Distracting ourselves may take all the willpower we can muster, but it is well worth stopping this unproductive rerunning of our thoughts, particularly at times when our thoughts cause us pain.

Many people have used this suggestion to distract themselves in dealing with their reactions to the loss of a loved one or to a traumatic event. Most of us think we have to rerun memories or feelings or issues related to distressing experiences in order to overcome them. I have found that this is not true, that repetitive, upsetting thoughts keep us upset, not resolved. Therefore, distracting ourselves can actually bring us relief.

NEGATIVE THINKING

Our constant attention on and talking about what hurts, what is wrong, what is missing, and what does not work is negative thinking. We all have minds that produce negative ideas. We think the worst, worry about terrible outcomes, and have fears and doubts. Since life is not perfect or problem-free, we cannot help but be prone to this kind of self-torture. The problem is not that we have such thoughts or feelings but that we *believe* whatever ideas go through our minds, that we embrace them, and then are overpowered by them. We think we are preparing ourselves for life's eventualities by thinking the worst, but all we are doing is making ourselves miserable.

Negative thinking causes us not only to suffer over unwanted or unpleasant circumstances of the moment but also to imagine such circumstances indefinitely into the future. If we have a fever or another disturbing physical problem, we think we will always be sick. If we are lonely, we imagine we will always be alone. If we are suffering grief over a loss, we believe our sorrow is interminable. We forget that nothing remains the same as it is today, that nothing is forever. However, most of us allow our feelings to dominate us and our experience of living, so that when we are sick or lonely or sad we cannot conceive of feeling satisfied with life.

The key is knowing that our feelings are temporary, unless we hang on to them or keep expressing or expanding upon them. With this understanding we can simply notice and respond to our feelings as they arise and then let them go as a momentary life experience. Not paying attention to our feelings, not sweeping them into our lives and embellishing them, may seem unimaginable or impossible, mainly because we have never done otherwise. How different our experience of living can be if we say to ourselves, "I feel sad," and continue to act in the present. We can avoid obsessive or negative thinking by picking up an interesting book to read or painting or mopping the floor or delving wholeheartedly into some other activity. Again, consciously distracting ourselves is a useful release from obsessing and negativity and from our other self-tortures as well.

WORRY

Worry is a popular form of negative thinking and self-torture. All of us worry, a little or a lot. We worry about war, and we worry about what to wear. We worry about having enough money, and we worry about having enough time. We worry about the past, the present, and the future. If something terrible happens, we worry that something worse will occur. Our worries encompass both our serious concerns and the smallest details of our everyday lives. Anything in life can be a source of worry for us.

Although it does not serve us to worry, many of us think worrying somehow enables us to cope or prepares us for unexpected eventualities. This is not true, for we cannot accurately predict or prepare for how life will proceed. Thus, worry is simply another habitual and debilitating mental activity, a self-torture that aids and resolves nothing.

Breaking the worry habit and other habits: How do we stop worrying? We need to see worrying as a habit, an entrenched habit. To successfully break any habit takes discipline and awareness. Primarily we need to commit ourselves to stop, which means to promise, no matter what, to let go of worrying. We need to take a firm stand, otherwise we can easily slide back into old, insidious ways.

Establishing the ongoing discipline not to indulge in worry when we are tempted may be the most difficult aspect of breaking this habit. Most of us have no experience in saying "No!" to our thoughts, so the idea of stopping any thoughts may seem absurd at first. Of course, worry will arise from time to time. Each time a worried thought appears, we must assert ourselves and say, "No! I'm not going to play with these thoughts." Then we may also need to distract ourselves by changing our environment or getting into some kind of involving activity.

If we say "no" to our thoughts again and again, ultimately we will learn to successfully manage or even eliminate our worrying habit. I have often had the thought that various loved ones would die in a car crash, since my brother died that way. I refuse to let that idea have too much importance, and I won't let worry consume me. Whenever that thought comes up, I quickly let it go.

All of us naturally give weight to our thoughts, and sometimes we will forget that our thoughts are just thoughts; sometimes we will believe what we think. At those times we will need to lovingly put ourselves back on track by remaking our promise to quit thinking this way. We may have to remake our promise many times over. However, we will feel very powerful when we do not indulge in habitual thoughts. This method can be effective in helping to break any of our self-torturing habits.

COMPLAINING

Because complaining is so common among us, it is a self-torture of which we are usually unaware. So frequent and automatic are our objections to our lives that we do not notice that we are complaining about the weather, the political situation, our bodies, each other, and endless other topics. Even though we may tune out or numb ourselves to our own and other people's objections, for many of us life is one big complaint.

Passive and ineffective, our complaints act as helpless stabs at injustices or disappointments and alter or further nothing. As a result, our complaints serve as self-torture, a kind of self-victimization. That we see life as something being done to us, something out of control, that we see ourselves as bystanders rather than designers of our lives, accounts in great measure for the extent of our complaining. Like treading water, complaining is an activity that keeps us in the same place for a long time.

We express our objections to life instead of taking any action to shift things. Consequently, our complaints serve to maintain our helplessness, our victim stance. Complaining depletes our energy and takes the heart out of our satisfaction. In fact, complaining can keep us interminably stuck with exactly what we think we do not want. It may be that we complain in order not to have to take the necessary steps to gain our own fulfillment.

Dealing with our complaints: An interesting experiment might be to notice how often we complain, or to notice in partnership with another person how much each of us complains. We might even list all of our complaints. Afterward we could examine our lists to see what we are willing to accept and what we intend to act upon to change. In this way we could begin to use our complaints as stepping stones to action. We may only be inclined to act on a small percentage of our complaints, which is fine as long as we are willing to let go of torturing ourselves with our remaining complaints.

Our objections to life may be valid. However, there are more satisfying ways of dealing with life than complaining. An effective alternative to consider is that we stop resisting life and accept things as they are, that we surrender to life. For instance, if the weather is hot, it is hot. No amount of complaining will alter that. If our partner is withdrawn right now, our partner is just withdrawn right now. Accepting, allowing life to be as it is, can afford us great peace of mind and ease of living, both the antidote for and the antithesis of self-torture.

FEAR

Fear is a natural reaction. Beyond real fear for our own survival, our biggest fears are rejection, loss, failure, and the unknown.

Sometimes fear warns and protects us, such as when we are driving too fast or walking down a dark street alone. More often fear is another kind of negative thought that we embrace, for, in essence, we literally scare ourselves with our own thoughts. Most of us think our fears are real, and so we let fear stop us. We allow ourselves to be victimized and controlled by our fears instead of letting them pass by like the varied scenery along a highway. When we embrace fear, fear controls us. That's self-torture!

Since we cannot eliminate fear from our lives, we need to have a successful relationship with fear. Most important is that we not let our fears dominate our actions, that we not be stopped by fear. The cure for fear is to push through the activity that frightens us, if we can. For we can discover that we can be afraid and do it anyway. Pushing through fear can stretch us, expand us, and truly enhance our lives. Many of us have become successful public speakers, even though we were initially afraid to confront an audience. Relationships, job promotions, sports, or daring activities like mountain climbing or roller-coaster riding are all the more exciting when we supersede, not erase, our fears. (We need to distinguish here between fear and terror. Terrified people are too upset, already feeling out of control, and should not be be pushed to act.)

We naturally experience fear in response to real danger or after traumatic events like a loss, fire, or accident. This is not self-torture but rather a natural protective mechanism operating in us. However, severe, immobilizing fear that is not connected to life-threatening events is not natural and may require the help of a qualified psychiatrist or psychotherapist to uncover its source and to help restore our power over our own lives.

GUILT OR REMORSE

Another classic form of torturing ourselves is guilt, which is self-blame, or the feeling that we have committed an offense or an error. We all make mistakes and fail on occasion. The problem is that rarely do we accept our error or offenses and simply dismiss them. Instead, most of us are quick to remind ourselves of wrongdoings and blame ourselves incessantly. We can continue to feel badly about our actions or the lack of them for a long, long time.

Often guilt is the result of our high expectations for ourselves and of how quickly we judge ourselves. We tend to feel badly over words we spoke or did not say and over actions we took or avoided. The extreme of such guilty, self-effacing behavior is the woman who bumped into a table and apologized to it!

Handling guilt: Even when we have acted very wrongly, obsessive guilt or remorse or constantly reminding ourselves of our offenses tortures us and resolves nothing. The healthiest response would be to admit we were wrong, take any necessary action, let the incident go, and not repeat the offense. If we expressed cruel words or acted thoughtlessly, we can ask to be forgiven. We can admit, "I was wrong, and I am sorry." We also need to forgive ourselves. "Forgiveness" is addressed more deeply later in chapter 22.

REGRET

Another form of self-torture, regret, is rampant among us. The Merriam-Webster Dictionary defines regret as "distress of mind on account of something beyond one's power to remedy." We have endless regrets. We regret our behaviors, incidents from the past, things done or not done, dreams achieved or not achieved. We look back on the road not taken as if we made a mistake, as if we should have functioned some other way. We constantly examine the past, and then we want to rewrite or alter the script, as if we could change the outcome. Our regrets leave us frustrated and unhappy.

In our relationships, we regret words unspoken, like "I love you," and the words already said, like "I hate you." We regret our actions. We are sorry for what we do, for our outbursts or out-of-control moments, for our ineffective or childish behaviors, and for what we did not do, the omissions in our actions. Nonetheless, every one of us acts childishly or ineptly or inappropriately sometimes.

Many of us believe that our regrets foster self-improvement and enable us to awaken to the errors of our ways. I say this is rare. More often we use our regrets for obsessing and punishing ourselves, not to improve ourselves. William, a retired successful businessman, keeps himself miserable with regrets. Much of his conversation centers on his regrets over past incidents and how he would now alter earlier life events. Poignantly, shortly before she died, his wife asked to be cremated. He didn't want to comply, but he did as she asked. Afterward William regretted that he had agreed to her cremation, that he hadn't simply buried her. For weeks his regrets consumed him as he shared his self-torture with anyone who would listen.

Regretting serves no useful purpose, except as self-torture. The strongest panacea for regret is to accept ourselves exactly as we are with all of our attributes and limitations. We must let go of regrets that we are not thin or blue-eyed or twenty years younger or an astronaut. If we see that we erred, we must forgive ourselves and let it go. We need to remember that we always do the best we can at any given moment, even though it may not look that way in hindsight. We must accept that there is no way to rewrite life. What is, is—period.

Releasing regrets: The following is a way of looking at and completing our regrets. First, we should take as much time as is necessary to list as many sentences as come to mind that would begin with the words "I regret," expressing anything that fits into this category, past or present. Then study the list. We should check each item on our lists to see if there is any action to be taken to complete it. If there is, we should write down specifically what that action would be and the date by which we will have completed it. For those regrets for which there are no actions to be taken, we must consciously let go now and forgive ourselves and whoever else is involved. All of us may secretly harbor regrets without realizing it, and so this is a useful exercise to do periodically. Releasing ourselves from regrets can give us renewed energy and zest for life.

Tragically, we often make ourselves miserable under the guise of supporting ourselves or helping ourselves to grow. Self-tortures are often old habits that we have unknowingly embraced, as if these methods would help us resolve or solve problems. We automatically trap ourselves in obsessive thinking, complaining, worry, and fear out of habit. Likewise, we have learned to blame ourselves and not forgive ourselves and thus we have become imprisoned in guilt and regret.

We can, if we choose, free ourselves from these forms of suffering. We can learn to stop, to say "no," to distract ourselves from our thoughts, and to forgive ourselves for our mistakes. We have the power to end our self-tortures now. Another habit that does not serve us is "withholding ourselves," which is discussed in the next chapter.

•14•

WITHHOLDING OURSELVES

It is impossible for a man to be cheated by anyone but himself.

RALPH WALDO EMERSON

A major source of our suffering in life is that we withhold ourselves from our lives, our experiences, and our relationships. Withholding or suppressing ourselves is a habit that actually occurs in epic proportions among us; most of us hold back, reserve, deny, or conceal at least part of ourselves. Even though we may be unaware that we do it, our withholding is often the source of our deadness, resignation, dissatisfaction, loneliness, and disappointment in life.

Withholding is a great killer of relationships. Not an instant killer, it is slow and insidious, like a poison that we inject a little at a time, building up to a lethal dose. Concealing and protecting ourselves and others, we deaden ourselves a little at a time and gradually cut off any possibilities for closeness. As we allow less and less of ourselves to be known, we feel shut off from others. Eventually we feel isolated and resentful. Unfortunately, we do not remember that we ourselves are the source of these feelings.

Linda came to me for therapy because she had "turned off" sexually from her husband, whom she loved and with whom she otherwise had a good relationship. Unaware of the source of the problem, she wanted to recover her lost sexual desire. I told her I had a suspicion as to what was wrong and asked if she was willing to clear up the problem in one hour of therapy. (Sometimes people come to a therapist for an ongoing relationship, or for some other reason, and are unwilling to let go of problems so quickly.)

After Linda said she was willing to resolve this in one hour, I gave her a pile of paper and a pen. I told her this was an experiment for her eyes only and asked her to write down anything she was not telling her husband. She wrote and wrote, ending up with three pages of notes. I suggested that this in itself represented how much of herself she was holding back from her husband. I asked her if she was willing to go home and talk with him about the things she had written down. She hesitated only briefly. Once she saw the price she was paying for holding back, that she had deadened herself, she was actually eager to open up communication with her husband. I never saw Linda again, but she wrote me a letter some weeks later saying that her sexual desire had returned and that her marriage was better than ever. Like Linda, many of us hold back a little or forget to say something, or decide to withhold, and don't notice it until we experience some serious consequence like lethargy or sexual deadness or disinterest in loved ones. Even then, we usually don't know that the cause of these symptoms is our suppressing of ourselves.

We tend to scare ourselves into silence. We usually withhold communication because of fears or concerns about the consequences of expressing ourselves. Dominated by our fears and other considerations, we elect what looks like the easier path—to be closed off or isolated from loved ones, consequently missing out on love, aliveness, and closeness. Probably the most serious consequence of withholding ourselves is that we remain strangers to those we love.

Chances are that each of us withholds ourselves somewhere or in some circumstances, although we may not be aware of it. Few of us feel free to be the same person in each of our relationships—the same with our spouse, parents, children, boss, colleagues, friends, neighbors, and strangers. Instead we often act like a chameleon, always changing our colors and trying to fit in with each person. This means we shape or alter our behaviors or words and we feel free to tell more to some people than to others. This takes enormous effort. In contrast, if we were the same with each person we encountered, we could be more natural, relaxed, authentic, and expressed.

STYLES OF WITHHOLDING

In order for us to see what up to now may be an unconscious pattern, several examples follow to demonstrate situations and styles of withholding. First, Joan married Karl, a man with definite likes and dislikes, a man who said "no" to much of life. In order to please him and to have his acceptance of her ideas, Joan would preselect whatever she told Karl. The more she was careful and selective in communicating, the more stilted she became. She finally sought psychotherapy because of her inability to express herself at all with Karl anymore.

Tom grew up thinking men are supposed to take charge and make life easy for their wives, that he should manage everything and not share his troubles. When faced with bankruptcy, he felt panic and withdrew more and more from his wife, June. In response, June felt rejected and hurt. Tom almost lost her before he dared say how scared and inadequate he felt.

Susan developed a crush on her husband's best friend. She began to feel tired and tense all day and sleepless at night. When through therapy she realized the source of her symptoms, she chose to stay physically distressed rather than to risk her husband's possible rejection if he knew the truth about her secret crush. As many of us do, Susan opted for harmony regardless of the cost, and she avoided resolving her feelings.

After Alice married Bill, she bought nothing for herself lest he get angry at her, like her father had, for being a spendthrift. She never discussed this with Bill. Three martyred years into marriage, Alice noticed herself desiring other men. Her withholding of her own wants and needs led her to cut herself off from Bill.

Joe was preoccupied with suspicions about his girlfriend, Nancy, seeing other men behind his back. Rather than tell her and risk looking foolish or risk her rejection, he drank several beers every evening after work to numb himself to his feelings. Ultimately, they ended their relationship because Nancy found Joe so unavailable and worried that he was an alcoholic.

These typical scenarios demonstrate that we withhold ourselves automatically under a wide range of circumstances. We hide our true feelings and end up with bewildering behaviors or symptoms or reactions, often as a result of our concealment. We wonder why our relationships deteriorate; we do not see that our holding back is the source of many of our difficulties and problems with one another.

THE ANTIDOTE TO WITHHOLDING: COMMUNICATION

The means to combating our withholding is to be authentic, to reveal rather than to conceal ourselves. It is not enough to say, "tell the truth," for that expression may trigger ambivalent feelings, fears, or doubts. All of us have experienced people who have used the so-called truth to hurt. I remember a couple, both psychologists, who used to hurtfully label and diagnose each other under the guise of telling the truth. She labeled him "passive-aggressive," and he called her "hysterical" and "narcissistic." How many people criticize under the guise of "I'm just saying this for your own good?" We learn to not trust each other's "truth" as a result. Our fear of the power of words—that words damage or destroy—is one justification for persistently withholding ourselves.

Speaking responsibly—telling the truth: Because we are all prone to having ulterior motives behind our words, we need to distinguish between telling the truth to damage or manipulate and telling the truth to express ourselves and complete something. Speaking responsibly is speaking for and of ourselves and opens communication. This is a very tricky distinction, for we invariably want our words to have some impact or influence on the other person. Usually we speak to cause a change of behavior or attitude in someone else rather than for the sake of self-expression and the internal freedom that such expression affords us. We have not learned to speak so as to simply clear up or resolve feelings, problems, or disagreements.

The saying "The truth shall set you free" has great power in it, since speaking the truth relieves us and makes understanding and intimacy possible. In contrast, in expressing only our opinions or judgments we are likely to feel shut down. Unfortunately, whatever is the truth often gets lost for us when we swallow our feelings. Once we are willing to tell the truth, we can begin to speak and the words will come to us. We will probably discover then that our truth is just a simple statement like "I am hurt" or "I am afraid."

Speaking responsibly—saying "I": A key to expressing ourselves responsibly is to communicate from "I" instead of "you." Our revealing ourselves might begin with a statement like "I am hurt," "I do not like," "I am disappointed," "I'm afraid that," "I didn't tell you," or "I want you to know." By itself, saying "I" can transform our communications. In other words, pointing a finger at ourselves when we speak instead of pointing a finger at another is responsible speaking.

Speaking responsibly—having purpose: What we intend to accomplish out of our speaking, the purpose of communication or self-revelation, will affect the results. Speaking in order to hurt, cajole, or manipulate does not open communication. The purposes for expressing the truth are to open communication, to expand our relationship with ourselves and others, and to finish with or complete a moment, memory, feeling, or experience we are having. Completeness is gained by expressing and then letting go of a thought or feeling once and for all. In relationships, as in so many aspects of life, completion generates satisfaction.

Speaking responsibly—having compassion: When we communicate with compassion and consideration for the other person as a worthwhile and trustworthy being, we are free to reveal ourselves without having to worry about damaging the other person in the process. Sometimes we simply have to choose to trust someone else, to create an atmosphere for communication. If we completely disregard the other and are simply intent upon unloading our feelings or ideas, chances are that our communication cannot succeed in resolving or completing anything.

"DUMPING"

Irresponsibly loading our every reaction on another person is not telling the truth, but rather is more appropriately called "dumping." In not expressing ourselves directly at the moment, many of us save up our thoughts and feelings to be expressed on some future occasion. Saving up old thoughts and feelings can be like saving garbage, and dumping is like vomiting, an automatic release of the old contents of our innards. It is not honest and open communication.

Forms of dumping—irresponsible communications—are blaming, shaming, and manipulating. We blame the other person by pointing our finger in their direction, which is evident in beginning our communications with "you" instead of "I." We may manipulate by being nasty, sarcastic, punitive, and self-righteous. Just loading down another person with our opinions or judgments of them can be a form of dumping, like the two psychologists who call each other names by using psychiatric diagnoses.

We can easily distinguish the truth from dumping by the effect our words have on the people around us. Truth usually frees people to experience further openness and loving feelings, to feel good. In contrast, dumping usually wreaks havoc in our relationships, for nothing is forwarded. Dumping doesn't open communication or create intimacy; people do not feel good afterward.

SUCCESSFULLY RELEASING FEELINGS

Dumping can feel like a satisfying purge, and sometimes we may need to unload our thoughts, feelings, reactions, or ideas. Since this does not further our relationships, we can use our time by ourselves for this purpose. As odd as this idea may sound at first, talking aloud to imaginary people or situations, instead of facing off with the real ones, allows us to voice *any* inner thoughts in any manner we wish. We do not have to worry then about hurting anyone else with our words, and so speaking aloud to ourselves can be cathartic and completing. This can also serve as a rehearsal or clearing ground for future communications, which might free us to speak more responsibly when the opportunity arises.

UNCOVERING WITHHOLDS

Whenever we don't know if we are withholding, we need to ask ourselves, "What am I not saying right now?" or "What am I withholding?" and to think of resentments, appreciations, hurts, sorrows, regrets, and the like we have in regard to specific people in our lives. We can write down whatever comes up, just as Linda did in the therapy described at the beginning of this chapter. We need to sit down and examine any or all of our relationships, looking for whatever it is that we are not saying. Chances are that we will notice unspoken words in all of our relationships because most of us habitually withhold ourselves everywhere without realizing it. Once we see what needs to be said, we should say it. If we can, we should say all of it.

There is much to be learned about ourselves from an exercise like this, and whatever we discover, whatever insights we have into ourselves, can be useful for enhancing our relationships. Some of us will discover that we are habitual withholders, that there is something we do not say in every one of our relationships. We may see a theme to our withholding, so that unexpressed in every relationships is, for example, our resentments. We may notice that we do not express our love, that we assume our intimates know without being told that we love them. We may uncover tightly guarded opinions or attitudes that were suppressed. It is not unusual to be selective, to be more open with some people than others. We may see how careful we are with particular people, like our parents or our spouse, or that we are more open with one sex than another. We may see that we opt for peace at any price, or that we are "nice" no matter what, or that we want to be liked more than we want to express ourselves.

Remember the purpose of communication is to express ourselves so that we can be complete or free of whatever we said. Incompletions keep us mired in the past, struggling endlessly with the same issues, unavailable for the present. Sometimes even after we express ourselves feelings persist because we are not heard. Completing communications is not the responsibility of the other person, for he or she may never "get" us. More important is that we pay attention to our own feelings, that we understand and accept ourselves. As much as we may want to be heard, the other person's responses are not as important as our own letting go, our own releasing of old thoughts or feelings. Once we discover old ideas and feelings persisting, we can take the opportunity now to let all that past go once and for all.

COMPLETING WHAT IS INCOMPLETE

We know that we are incomplete when an idea or feeling repeats itself, or when we feel unsatisfied in a relationship or in our communications with another. Dissatisfaction is an indicator that something more needs to be done in examining, revealing, and expressing ourselves, either directly with the other person or for our own information. When we discover what we have withheld, we can examine each withheld communication to see if we can let it go and be complete with it right now or if we need to tell another person directly.

If we discover that something on our list needs to be expressed directly to someone else, we then have to look at whether or not we are willing to do so. A good question to ask ourselves is "Will this communication forward our relationship, or would it be dumping?" For now we can distinguish more easily what is useful to express to another.

Having our intention and attention on communicating clearly and responsibly makes a big difference in the outcome. If we communicate intending to be complete, we will naturally speak in such a way as to cause that to happen. Being complete is actually a stand we can take to let go (of whatever the item is) right now and for always.

EXPRESSING OURSELVES IN WRITING

There are times when we feel incomplete or confused, and we cannot tell another our feelings or thoughts directly. Then a useful tool can be writing a letter that we do not send as an opportunity to express ourselves. We can use the letter to say whatever needs to be said in whatever form we want to say it, writing until we feel we have said everything we needed to say. Expressing ourselves on paper can be a very satisfying means of release.

Once such a letter is written, it probably should be destroyed. What is of value in writing the letter is the opportunity for our own personal release. Sometimes we become so enamored with our own words that we forget their potency in wanting to share them with the addressee. Now that we understand the distinction between communicating and dumping, we can select exactly what to say to enhance the relationship with another person.

STAYING CURRENT IN OUR COMMUNICATIONS

Few of us are so conscious in our relationships that we are always fully up-to-date with our communications, fully truthful and expressed with everyone in our lives. Periodically stopping to clear out any of our current withholds can enhance our relationships and give us a sense of the direction we need to take. This is a way to be fully responsible for ourselves, our communications, and our relationships.

Several couples I know have a commitment always to tell each other the truth, which they attest is the source of their having long lasting and satisfying intimate relationships. One of these couples never says good-bye in the morning without knowing they are each clear with one another. Another never says good night if there is anything between them or in the way. Great intimacy is possible when we and our partners trust each other so completely that we always fully and openly express ourselves with one another. There is enormous freedom and satisfaction in that kind of intimacy. Revealing ourselves fully, being authentic, is one of the great secrets of being satisfied, complete, and open to life. This is available to any of us if we stop withholding ourselves.

Another kind of withholding of ourselves that is equally self-defeating is when we live halfheartedly. This is something many of us do without realizing it and is addressed in the next chapter.

• 15 •

LIVING HALFHEARTEDLY

The tragedy of life is what dies inside a man while he lives.

ALBERT SCHWEITZER

L ife's hurts, sorrows, and disappointments are a primary
motivation to stop living full out, to live halfheartedly.
Sometimes after we confront upsetting events, we do not want
to try again and risk facing another failure or disappointment.
Drained of courage and energy, we cut ourselves off from life
and live halfheartedly.

Halfhearted living has several distinguishing characteristics.
The most obvious are a vague sense of dissatisfaction and a lack
of enthusiasm for life. In simplest terms, halfheartedness shows
when we say "no" a lot to life. It is living in resignation, seeing
life as full of impossibilities instead of possibilities, seeing no
room for changes or alterations or anything new to occur. We
simply feel stuck with life as it is; we go through the motions of
living.

REACTING TO UPSETTING EVENTS

Our halfheartedness can be a reaction to a loss, crisis, or trauma
in our lives. We may shut down or pull energy out of our lives

as a result of any painful experience. Catherine sought therapy, complaining of deadness and lack of enthusiasm for life. She was "going through the motions of life, but not living." When I asked when she first noticed her deadness, she said, "Since September," eight months before. I asked what had happened then, and she told me rather nonchalantly that she had lost all her money because of a bad investment. Still she was bewildered by her deadness, fearfulness, and withdrawal from life, for before that she had been happy and enthusiastic. Although she said she had no feelings about it now, she remembered she was upset at the time and felt stupid that she had made such a mistake. Innocently, she mentioned that when she found out about her financial loss, she kept saying to herself, "Life will never be the same for me." This statement became a self-fulfilling prophecy, for she made it true by not living fully from that moment on. It was also true that the loss of money dramatically changed her life-style, for she moved from a luxurious home to a studio apartment and now had to work for a living.

What Catherine did is not as unusual as we would like to think. As mentioned earlier, in the dire moments of our lives, without necessarily being aware of it, we make statements or promises to ourselves that can potently affect all the rest of our lives. Usually these statements are promises to restrict or control ourselves, for we often want to contract and close up after a bad experience. Once we do close up this way, we may not remember why.

UNCOVERING OUR SELF-FULFILLING PROPHECIES

If we will take the time to recall our trauma and run it through in our minds in detail, our "prophecy" will usually become obvious. We should do this at a time when we can have quiet and privacy and as much time as we need to look backward. These are the key questions to ask ourselves: When did this feeling (of deadness, disappointment, distrust, dissatisfaction, or sadness) begin? What happened then? What did I say to myself about it? Or what promises did I make then? Chances are that we will discover that in some form or another we said, "I will never again" or "I will always." When we were upset and unaware, we most likely took strong stands that are affecting our lives today, stands that specifically generated our future behavior and became prophecies.

Catherine saw that she was perpetuating her "prophecy" from the time she lost her money. Before she could let it go, she had to relinquish her guilt and forgive herself for making a mistake. Interestingly, the mistake she really felt she made was in putting her money into someone else's hands and not following it closely. She blamed herself for not being responsible for her money, and that is what she had to forgive in order to become fully open to her life again. I had her express her forgiveness fully by saying aloud to herself, "I forgive you." This was hard for her to say, for we resist the idea of forgiving ourselves. However, once Catherine did so, she was free to fully engage in her life again. She promised she would stay fully alive and that she would create a satisfying life for herself from now on. Several months later she called to tell me she was still keeping her promise.

LIVING WITH MINIMUM EFFORT

Halfheartedness always generates dissatisfaction, yet many of us persist in living halfheartedly much of the time. Early on in life we learned to get by with minimum effort and minimum expression of ourselves. We discovered how to always hold something of ourselves back. Most of us began living halfheartedly long ago. Hurt, disappointed, or humiliated when we expressed ourselves as children, or when we were confronted with early failure or rejection, we decided to close ourselves off. "How little can I say or do?" became a game we played with the world, for we determined how to do that limited amount and no more and thus escape notice. Already familiar with that negative mode, when a crisis or upsetting event occurs we simply pull back more and give out less.

Habitually doing our least but no longer aware of our restriction, we wonder why we usually feel vaguely dissatisfied. We do not know any more that we are curbing ourselves. We may not remember the beginning of our holding back. Over time some of us have simply felt worn down by life; we go on as if living full out and fully open is not worth the effort anymore. The number of hours each day that we sit around and watch television may be an indicator of how little we are engaged in really living today.

WAITING INSTEAD OF ACTING UPON OUR LIVES

Another chronic source of our halfhearted living is that we wait for life to present itself to us, instead of creating life ongoingly. Many of us have a tendency to wait. We live halfheartedly now, waiting and hoping for a substantial reason to come fully alive again at some future time. Sometimes we imagine if only we had the right job or the perfect love partner or a sense of our true purpose, then we would open ourselves totally to life. Often we act like Sleeping Beauty in the fairy tale, waiting for someone else, our special prince or princess, to awaken us to life. We may not all expect to be rescued by another, but we wait for some special signal or dimension of life to show itself to us before we will completely give *all* of ourselves. Some of us wait our whole lives.

PROTECTING OURSELVES

Self-protection is another purpose of our halfheartedness. We are so intent on not being disappointed or hurt again that we cut off our aliveness. We are afraid to risk failure. We dread playing life full out and then not succeeding. Holding ourselves back, we imagine we can minimize some of the risk that life is. This method usually backfires since life always presents risks, whether we live wholeheartedly or not.

BEING COMFORTABLE INSTEAD OF BEING CHALLENGED

Our halfheartedness is also based on our natural propensity to be comfortable rather than living at risk and being uncomfortable. We opt for life to be easy rather than challenging. For that reason we stay in unsatisfying jobs and deadening relationships, as they are familiar and undemanding. Since comfort taxes us minimally, we can coast through our lives both unstressed and unstretched. Unfortunately, we do not feel very alive when we are coasting.

TRANSFORMING HALFHEARTEDNESS TO WHOLEHEARTEDNESS

Our chronic halfheartedness can be transformed once we see it and once we are willing to be fully alive again. Transforming our halfheartedness requires a commitment to aliveness. Such a move might be uncomfortable and jolting, for relinquishing our halfhearted behaviors means giving up some favorite entrenched habits. We would have to give up hanging back and avoiding people or new experiences. We would no longer get away with not speaking up or with saying "no" to something new.

Wholehearted living is more of an experiment, more of a surprise, and definitely more fun. To live wholeheartedly from now on is a conscious choice that we might rechoose daily. The key is that we need to commit ourselves to living full-out all of the time. It means giving up holding back, lying around, hiding from life. Instead we would be committed to stretching ourselves, to being challenged, to risking, and to being fully expressed. Wholehearted, we would say "Yes!" to life much more than "No!" or "I don't want to." Keeping a promise to ourselves to live fully might mean living at 100 percent effort, 100 percent of the time.

It is hard to suffer when we are fully alive! While halfhearted living tends to leave us feeling half asleep, living life full out requires that we be very awake, truly alive to every moment and all the possibilities life offers us. Vital and excited by life, we are bound to be satisfied.

• 16 •

GOING IT ALONE

I had a lover's quarrel with the world.

ROBERT FROST

Many of us think we must face life as adults alone, so we learn to function more and more as "loners" or "Lone Rangers," as solitary beings who tend to avoid needing or trusting other people. Functioning alone may be our idea of being "grown-up" and independent, but usually this is a defensive maneuver designed to protect us from being hurt or disappointed—again. Ironically, going it alone more often accentuates our pain.

In order to appear to be capable adults, we often take charge of our own survival with a vengeance. The force with which we trudge on independently through life may leave us deeply lonely and virtually starving for nourishment. Having to confront life's hurts alone makes them tougher, and yet many of us can't imagine an alternative. However, it is possible for us to reexamine our style of managing our lives so that we can have a choice of being alone or not.

THE SOURCE OF THE "LONER" STYLE

The "loner" style is usually born out of pain and disillusionment stemming from our earlier experiences. This style seems to be a reaction to our childhood, when we were helpless and literally needed other people to survive. Many of us despise that remembered helplessness and the frustration of being so needful, while others fear our attraction to succumbing to being taken care of and possibly being taken over by another again. Many of us were so hurt or disappointed by other people early in life that we grew up with the idea that we will only succeed more safely and more easily alone. Out of our childhood experiences, we decided that we will "never again" need people or rely on people or trust or be vulnerable or be "taken in by" people again. Our "never again" statements become self-fulfilling prophecies. Thus, we make it impossible to avail ourselves of other people's support.

OUR NEED FOR RELATIONSHIPS

Even though we have been hurt or disappointed before, we do not have to base the rest of our lives on those hurts. Relationships can be one of the most satisfying and sustaining aspects of life. Yet often this area is so fraught with conflict that we cut ourselves off from the exquisite sustenance that friendships and intimacy can provide. We deny ourselves the love and support that could enhance the quality of our lives. We hold ourselves back from contributing to others, and we fight against people contributing to us.

Because we do not avail ourselves of the opportunity of having expanded relationships and we do not share ourselves intimately with many others, we begin to believe we are alone in life. At one time or another most of us feel not just alone but virtually isolated or different from other people. When we have no one with whom we share ourselves, no intimacy, we miss seeing similarities and commonalities among us. With no feedback from others we live in our own private world, and tend to believe whatever we privately think. All alone, our perspective can be very limited and self-centered. When we live in isolation, life may seem very hard, very effortful and very unsatisfying.

Although we may protest the idea, we are social beings, designed to relate and communicate. A meaningful support system of people, an abundance of people on whom to rely, to be intimate with, and to be supported by, makes our lives rich with possibilities. Close friends can be a daily source of fulfillment as well as important mainstays for our rougher confrontations with life. Counting on other people and extending ourselves for others generates vitality and satisfaction.

BARRIERS TO INTIMACY

We believe we are separate and alone: Before we can see the possibilities of friendship, we need to examine our barriers to tolerating such deep communions with others. Our sense of aloneness is one of our barriers. Because we cut ourselves off from and maintain fairly superficial contact with other people, we begin to believe we are separate and alone amidst hundreds of people in our everyday surroundings. We convince ourselves that no one else could understand how we feel. Of course we tell no one about ourselves, so we are not understood.

We think one person to love is fulfilling enough: Many of us settle for just that. This is another way we limit ourselves—we devote all of our time to just one other being, neglecting everyone else. For some of us it takes all the energy we can muster to let in just that one other person. Sadder still, some of us cannot even allow ourselves to be close with the one person with whom we have chosen to share our life.

We lie and say we do not need other people: Hurt before, we justify denying ourselves companionship with the idea that we need no one. We are afraid to impose and afraid to look needy or greedy, so we pretend we have no needs.

We are too wary to receive: We are uneasy about letting others into our lives in any personal or confidential way, and we find it particularly difficult to need anything from others. We may simply never allow other people to contribute to our well-being at all, ever. If someone wants to contribute to us, we either think something is wrong with us or that other people must be trying to dominate, manipulate, or "con" us. Even though our mistrust and our managing alone are burdensome, many of us would rather protect our vulnerability and suffer alone.

We are unwilling to trust: Out of being hurt or disappointed by other people in the past, we make a decision not to trust again. We are so busy looking backward to avoid having fate repeat itself that we miss looking forward toward nourishing ourselves with other, possibly new people. We are loners.

We are lazy: We are unwilling to expend the energy it takes to have and maintain close friendships since for many of us having friends seems like hard work. We imagine that making plans, telephoning, or writing letters demands too great an effort. Our jobs and families are so all-consuming that we think we have little left to invest in those outside our intimate circle. In resisting friendships lest they drain us, we overlook the possibility of being expanded or energized by others. We also miss experiencing how satisfying it is to contribute to someone else.

We have the misconception that "grown-up" means "alone": We mistakenly translate the adult qualities of being independent and able into being separate and apart, which are not the same thing. The implication of needing others, or of just having relationships with other people, is that we ourselves are then not able. This establishes our self-enforced isolation from other people. As a result, we typically face our difficult confrontations with life alone because "grown-ups" do not ask for company or assistance. Whether we force ourselves to act or we procrastinate or we avoid the situation altogether, the task seems all the more difficult.

THE POSSIBILITIES OF FRIENDSHIP

Having company can make all the difference in the ease with which we get potentially difficult tasks done, like buying or fixing a car, finding a better job, going to the doctor, sorting important papers, or attending a funeral. Having a friend along is not a statement of our incompetency, but rather of our ability to be nourished and supported.

A friend can be an incomparable support. Perhaps the greatest service a friend can offer is to remind us of who we are when we forget. With a friend we can express and release our innermost thoughts, fears, dreams, and sorrows, where our inner or private selves are most clearly captured and reflected back for us to see. A friend can lift us above our petty thoughts and self-criticisms. Left to our own devices, we usually have a distorted sense of ourselves. A good friend not only reflects back to us how we really show up in the world, our breadth and possibilities, but also can see aspects of us beyond what we see; he or she may know us better than we know ourselves.

There are also particular times in life when we would be wise to call on our friends to support us, perhaps with a daily telephone call or visit that would help us to face some difficult persisting problem or situation. When we or family members are ill or in trouble, when we are in the first throes of grief after a loss or trauma, a friend can listen, offer solace, advise, or simply serve as witness to our experience. A friend can lighten our load. Someone who can be with us when we are under stress is a great friend indeed.

Although we may worry about the burden or demands of friendship, the gift of our time and attention can make an enormous difference. Our reward is to know that we really contributed to another person's life. We may have to define our limits so that we do not feel resentful of or depleted by another's needs. Yet, most of us could manage a daily fifteen-minute telephone call if a friend needed us.

I have asked a lot of people who suffered serious problems in life what most helped them get through them. Over and over people told me their friends made the biggest difference in their coping. My clients and friends suffering from fatal illnesses all have said what eased the anguish of the diagnosis and the pain of the illness was the attention and love of their friends.

To make that kind of difference in the life of another person is truly satisfying and rewarding. Sometimes when a friend is in trouble we want to run away. We are afraid of confronting the worst or afraid that we are inadequate to the task at hand. To get through those moments, we need to draw on our courage and commitment to that other person. Ultimately those can be nourishing and satisfying times, times when we all grow the most.

I have been richly rewarded with friends. When I went home to the East Coast from California to be with my mother during the last weeks of her life, my friend Ellen and I arranged in advance that I would call Ellen daily at 5:00 p.m. Those telephone calls were the single greatest gift that Ellen could ever have given me, for I had the opportunity to cry, share, demonstrate my strength, get advice, and be understood during that most difficult time. Ellen said she appreciated and respected herself more than ever before, for she saw her value as a support, as a friend.

When my father died nine months later, Ellen arranged for her family and her business to be handled so that she could come home with me for a week to attend the funeral and to help me close my parents' apartment, both dreaded tasks for me. Her companionship and love were an incredible support for me in a tough time, and Ellen's presence was a continual reminder of who I am. As a result I maintained myself through other people's grief, emotionalism, pity, advice, and patronization. We worked hard, and we even laughed together at times. What ahead of time appeared a horrendous confrontation was an unpleasant but manageable event.

Even if we have been functioning as loners up to now, we can bring friends into our lives. Once we are open to friendship, it is amazing how easily we can meet people. Four different times in my life, I moved to cities where I knew no one. I met people in my apartment building, job, the supermarket, classes, the library, and at parties. Just the other day, I made a new friend at a wedding. People to know are all around us in the world if we but open ourselves to them.

Friends can be a great antidote to suffering; they are one of the most valuable resources available to us on the planet. We do not have to face everything in our lives alone. The next chapter elaborates on a different aspect of this same theme, which is "Denying Our Needs."

• 17 •

DENYING OUR NEEDS

This above all: to thine own self be true . . .
SHAKESPEARE, *HAMLET*

O ur greatest power over our lives comes from our ownership or our embracing of all that we are, our accepting
that we need love and to be loved, to be nurtured, to express
ourselves, to be noticed and acknowledged and more. Yet, most
of us do not accept these needs in ourselves. It may take courage,
and we may need help learning to do so. Invariably our needs
are all the more evident to us after we suffer a hurt or trauma.
If we cannot accept and respond to our needs, especially during
distressing times, our recovery will be slow or even stalemated.

What stops us from accepting our needs is that most of us
seem to be embarrassed or even ashamed to have any emotional
requirements. Just the word "need" seems to have a negative
connotation for many of us. We often hold "needs" as bad or
childish or as reflecting emotional problems, so we do our best
to deny or repress or conceal our needs from ourselves and
everyone else. However, what we try to bury usually does not
simply disappear, but most likely quietly persists without our
awareness of it. Then our concealed needs emerge, sometimes
in unexpected or embarrassing or disturbing ways. We suddenly

cry inappropriately, or we are hurt by something insignificant, or we hang on too tightly to someone who resents it. We talk too much or "show off." No matter how we try, we cannot run away from our needs. We would do best to face our needs head-on.

We accentuate our suffering when we disown our needs. Because we have the idea that as adults we should be finished with many of our emotional requirements, we hide from any emotional needs and cover them up with denials and pretenses. This is costly behavior because it alienates us from ourselves and our pain, causes problems in other areas, like our relationships, health, and vitality, and makes resolving painful experiences difficult, if not impossible.

We will have emotional needs forever. If we could learn to allow, accept, and find ways to satisfy our needs, life and the upsetting events in life would be so much easier to bear. No longer having to pretend or keep up our guard, we could find the means to support and empower ourselves to recover from and be complete with the traumatic times. Day-to-day life could be easier as well. Of all the needs we have, the need to be taken care of is the most persistent and often the hardest to accept.

THE NEED TO BE TAKEN CARE OF

Although we have many basic needs, the need to be taken care of is ever present and invariably causes us conflict. It is most obvious when we are hurting. This need usually distresses us, so we rarely satisfy it. We tend to deny it, run away from it, lie about it, distort it, and frustrate it. What we rarely do as adults is face it directly.

Most of us come into adulthood with a great deal of conflict and ambivalence in regard to having our needs met, particularly our dependency needs. Not only does the extended period of being taken care of in childhood ingrain in us a wish to be ongoingly nurtured, but also the disappointments from our childhoods set us up to avoid or distrust this need. As adults often we want to make up for what we missed as children, and are then disappointed. It is inevitable that somewhere in the many years of our childhoods we were not taken care of to our satisfaction. Some people were severely deprived of good parenting, and these people often have the hardest time dealing with their own needs. Besides that, all parents are bound to disappoint in some way, and little children can act like automatic "I want" machines who grasp for everything within reach. Children also distort with "If you love me, you would give it to me," the beginning of a confusion between need and love that may persist all of our lives.

Unavoidably disappointed in our childhoods, we develop several reactions to deny our original natural wish for nurturance. Our earlier experiences can leave us feeling very needy, yet most of us cover up that neediness. We may pretend we have no such needs as adults. We may be wary and distrustful of others and have difficulty in building intimate relationships. As described in the last chapter, we may take the stance of loners in life, acting as if we need no one. We may find covert ways to need others, like being sick a lot, talking too much, needing to be "center stage" all the time, or making enormous yet subtle demands on our friends and loved ones. Whatever form the denial of our dependency needs takes, we are apt to live with intense conflict between wanting to be taken care of and fearing that other people cannot or will not ever meet our needs.

INDIRECTLY MEETING OUR NEEDS

The most common indirect way to get our needs met is to take care of other people by being a caretaker—a mother, doctor, nurse, psychotherapist, or teacher. Our giving masks, but does not make up for, our feelings of deprivation or longing. A dramatic example of this were the welfare mothers I met years ago in my child-guidance work. Many of these women had one child after another but were starving for personal nourishment. Like many women in our society, they learned to deny their own needs for nurturing while growing up. Although these mothers were supposedly "sublimating" their needs by taking care of babies, the demands of many children left them even hungrier than they were before. Taking care of others only gives us the illusion that our own needs are being met or that we do not have needs of our own.

PROBLEMS THAT REFLECT OUR DENIAL OF OUR NEEDS

We can see evidence for our frustrated dependency needs everywhere—in our relationships with people, money, our health, our bodies, and even managing time. We cannot really hide from or deny our wish to be nurtured, for it is bound to reveal itself somewhere in our behavior, in how we get attention or in the covert ways we seek help.

For many of us health is the only area where we allow ourselves to be nurtured. Thus, we may develop physical symptoms or chronic illnesses that require the care of doctors or other helpers or the special attention of our loved ones. Most extreme was a woman who had a different type of surgery every year, a very disturbing way to have her emotional needs met. (More is said about this in chapter 21, "Our Bodies and Our Health.")

Our relationship with money reflects our mixed feelings about nurturing ourselves. We may have trouble earning money or saving money or keeping jobs because of our ambivalence about taking care of ourselves. Others of us manage money poorly, even to the point of putting ourselves into bankruptcy, because we are unwilling to be responsible for taking care of ourselves. In contrast, some of us need to have a lot of money as a statement of our independence from others.

Managing time is another area influenced by our ambivalent attitude toward our needs. Our difficulty in taking personal time for ourselves or managing our own time effectively is symptomatic of this ambivalence. The extreme is the workaholic, who totally denies his personal needs and never takes time off.

Our expectations of our relationships reflect our conflicts about needing one another and our earlier deprivations, as evidenced in the covert demands or expectations we place on others. We often expect our mates to give us what our parents gave or never gave. (It is also hard to give our children what we never got.) We may expect our partner to do all the driving or all the cooking. We may expect our partner to listen to us endlessly or to demonstrate his or her love in some other particular way. We are disappointed, often deeply disappointed, if he or she lets us down.

GAPS IN OUR INDEPENDENCE

Even though we may be very successful in life, we are often secretly unwilling to be fully independent, to manage all aspects of our lives well for ourselves. We leave gaps, for underneath it all we wish that someone else would do it for us. Typical is the competent business executive unable to boil an egg, or the woman who manages a home and several children and yet cannot fill out a simple business form or drive a car. When we claim incompetency or refuse to learn certain tasks, we cover up with other excuses. We will rarely admit that we do not do some task because of our wish to be taken care of by someone else. Both Robin Norwood's *Women Who Love Too Much* and Colette Dowling's *The Cinderella Complex* elaborate on this issue, particularly as it applies to women.

SUCCESSFULLY HANDING OUR NEEDS

The best way we can cope with our needs for nurturance is to reveal them, to admit them, and then to seek, if possible, to satisfy them. Seeing how our needs are thwarted or how we express our needs indirectly through illness and incompetency, for example, can be the first step to recognizing that we do have needs to be taken care of. After telling the truth and admitting our needs comes accepting and allowing needs as natural and human. Only then can we be free to have our needs met.

In being truthful about ourselves and our needs we can see what it would take for us to be nurtured. Then we can take action to fulfill our needs. We can directly ask for what we need and be aware of taking better care of ourselves. We can ask for a hug or help with a problem or time off for ourselves. Asking for what we want, leaving room for people to say "yes" or "no" in response, is freeing. Admitting our needs gives us the chance to have them met. Up to now most of us have been more adept at thwarting our needs than satisfying them, and so, for example, we may talk a lot and still long for something, or we put out a lot of energy or effort only to feel tired and unsatisfied. Satisfying our needs takes telling the truth and risking reaching out for or asking for what we really want.

Asking for what we want: One way to have our needs met is to ask for what we want specifically. Asking strengthens our ability to know what we want and to satisfy ourselves. In therapy, I have often given clients the exercise of allowing themselves to say "I want" often throughout the day in order to get in touch with their wants. "I want a glass of water" may have as much significance as "I want to be hugged." This seemingly simple exercise can open up a much deeper communion with ourselves.

Learning to ask in relationship with a partner is another kind of exercise. The first step would be to figure out what we want: a back rub, a quiet candlelit dinner, an hour of conversation to solve a problem, or time in bed to read to one another, for example. We can ask our partners or a friend for time, an hour or a day, to have exactly what we want, what we ask for directly. Then we can take turns with that other person and give to them what they ask of us. Giving each other what is asked for leads each person to feel fulfilled. Couples who have added this to their relationships have discovered whole new avenues for giving and receiving with one another and are more deeply satisfied as a result.

We can explore what might be nourishing for us that is now missing in our lives. The list of *Tools for Healing* in the chapter "Recovering Ourselves" is a good place to begin looking at what is nurturing. We can get pampered regularly in some satisfying way. We can ask for specific kinds of help or advice when we need it. We can be more open to having others contribute to us. Most of us seem to enjoy contributing a thousand times more than asking. Learning to allow our needs and to ask will totally alter our relationship with our needs.

In this section, we have addressed behaviors that contribute to our suffering in life, behaviors that are mostly habitual and out of our awareness. In the next section, we will look at particular areas of life where most people have difficulty and suffer, some of "The Arenas of Suffering."

· III ·

ARENAS OF SUFFERING

• 18 •

SEPARATING FROM
OTHER PEOPLE

Ah, when to the heart of man
Was it ever less than a treason
To go with the drift of things
To yield with a grace to reason,
And bow and accept the end
Of a love or a season?

ROBERT FROST

Loving and then letting go is one of the toughest lessons of life, a lesson every one of us confronts at some time. Relationships do not necessarily last forever. In fact, most relationships are limited in time; people die and people leave. We change our hearts or our minds or our interests in people. We grow and move on and sometimes leave people behind. Accepting that relationships change as a fact of life, not as a personal assault, would help us deal more successfully with separation and loss. Cultivating our ability to let go can be a most important step to easing and expanding our lives and to releasing us from suffering. This chapter examines our difficulty in separating from primary relationships.

Separating easily with a minimum of distress is a skill few of us learn, even though we all have a wealth of experience with endings and changes from birth onward. Separation and loss threaten us at our very roots, our survival. Our most primitive anxiety is that we will not survive after a separation, which makes facing partings and endings all the more complicated and difficult. As a result, our intimate relationships are often tinged with great need, and losing them seems a frightening and overwhelming prospect. We may cling to each other too tightly and yet be afraid to act or express ourselves with loved ones. We may demand too much or ask too little because we fear losing an intimate.

Divorce or separation is different from facing the death of a loved one. Sometimes divorcing or separating from living people seems harder because it is not as clear-cut or absolute as death. We may have to continue to relate to this person from whom we are parting, and our feelings can be more confused and ambivalent. We may experience more intense anger or rejection or failure in the breakup of a relationship. Others are sometimes less sympathetic or understanding than they might be if we were mourning a death or disaster in our lives.

We usually have strong and uncomfortable reactions to separating from one another. We may have fears, perhaps hidden fears, of rejection and loss or abandonment or desertion that are painfully realized when a relationship ends. We also fear the unknown, isolation, loneliness, neediness, or social ostracism. We do not want to have to face uncomfortable feelings like sorrow, regret, resentment, rage, and guilt. Perhaps hardest to face is feeling impoverished, inadequate, or depressed.

We may avoid separations at all cost because these reactions associated with separating seem so intolerable. We may stay in unsatisfying relationships or jobs. We may compromise how we behave, or we may suppress ourselves in order to keep someone else around. We can be too careful with one another. Tragically, we are often too afraid to risk speaking the truth with one another, even when the truth might enable us to resolve our problems. Many a marriage or friendship ends after too many feelings have been bottled up and unexpressed, sapping all aliveness in the relationship. As stated in the discussion of withholding ourselves, the habit of swallowing our feelings can destroy our relationships.

By avoiding separations we never learn to accept and allow the depths of emotion that embody the experience of letting go. We do not learn to tolerate sadness or anger or the many moments of emptiness in life, or discover that we all feel lonely and isolated at times regardless of our circumstances. We do not develop any ease in living with our reactions, and we lose confidence in our own resiliency and self-sufficiency. In avoiding tasting our emotions, we fail to discover that they are just a passing phase, not a permanent state.

Hence, most of us rarely allow for natural endings or directly express our good-byes. Instead, rather than something we initiate, letting go is usually imposed upon us by circumstances. This leads us to feel like victims whenever we confront separations in life.

Since our very survival seems threatened by having to part from one another, our behaviors in reaction to separating are defensive, sometimes crippling, and are among our most unsatisfying. To develop a deeper understanding of how we cope with change and separation and to open more possibilities for ourselves for the future, let us examine a variety of ways we separate from our intimate relationships.

UNSUCCESSFUL WAYS WE SEPARATE FROM RELATIONSHIPS

Denial: It is natural for us to wish to make the unpleasant disappear. For many of us our first reaction to any chance of separating from another is to deny it, to simply not see it. Confronting parting can seem so difficult, so unimaginable, that we attempt to block it out.

Often a client suffering the unwanted breakup of a relationship will say he or she had no warning. If true, both parties denied the seriousness of their problems or of their wish to separate. Sometimes the person who left gave no signals that he or she was unhappy, denying for the sake of the partner whatever misery preceded the breakup until it was impossible to hide those feelings any longer. More likely, the person who was left was unwilling to see signs that the relationship was in trouble. Even after a relationship is over, some people take years to unveil any awareness of the indicators that preceded an ending.

We repeatedly gloss over criticisms, doubts, differences, and disagreements in order to avoid conflict or confrontations that could lead to separating from one another. We tolerate and tolerate until one partner reaches a saturation point and decides to leave. As difficult as it is to take the responsibility of being the "leaver," it is often less painful than being the one left. As the one left, we tend to assume we are unworthy or at fault rather than examining the real causes for the dissolution.

The antidote to denial is expressing ourselves, sharing our dissatisfactions with as well as our appreciation of one another. We need to ask and speak about what's wrong and not shield the other person or ourselves from the truth. As uncomfortable as such openness may seem at first, it can enhance intimacy.

Although breaking through denial can seem frightening, it can be a great relief and might even save our relationships.

Delay: We put off dealing with issues that could upset a relationship, and we may put off the painful act of separating until some future time. Because our excuses for delay are often so reasonable, we may be unaware of our delaying tactics. We can be miserable in a marriage and still tell ourselves we must stay together because of the children, money, impracticalities of separating households, our families, or social disapproval. We convince ourselves that these reasons are more important than our aliveness or joy or satisfaction.

Our excuses for delay may also mask some serious anxieties about separating. Uncovering and examining these fears of loneliness, of failure or inadequacy, that render us immobile can give us a greater sense of personal power and can free us to be more effective with or without our relationship. Not examining issues and not acting keep us powerless.

A delaying couple I met socially, Pam and Doug, agreed that their marriage was ended but did not separate. They made no attempt to resolve their differences or to heal their relationship or be intimate, yet neither wanted to move from their house and children. They were at a stalemate, in separate bedrooms for three years. Admittedly unhappy together, neither was willing to risk detaching from their mutual dependency to go on alone until one of them found another partner and ended the stalemate.

Even though he was financially able and separate housing was available to him, for several years after college Mark lived with his parents, complaining incessantly about their faults. Mark represents those who have the hardest time separating from parents: those who felt most deprived. They stay, as if driven by the fantasy that eventually they will get the love they craved and missed. This never works. Delaying separation does not insure that our needs will be met. What we did not get, we did not get. We cannot fill in now what was missing in the past. Again, we have to admit what we missed, grieve, and release it to be free to create love newly today.

Partially separating: We sometimes maintain ourselves with one foot in and one foot out of a relationship. Some married people live totally separate lives, with separate bedrooms and separate friends, and simply share the same domicile. Marriages exist where one or both spouses is deeply involved with another partner, and yet divorce is never considered. People hold on to very unsatisfying relationships this way.

A similar case is the young person who has his own home yet spends more time in his parents' home or uses his parents' home for needs like laundry, meals, or receiving mail. The young person or his parents or both may be having difficulty separating from one another. Overprotective parents often create situations in which their children cannot easily generate independent lives. With this kind of crippling "support" system, we do not learn the courage to cope with living on our own.

Never separating: We all know children who never leave home or who live within walking distance in order to maintain daily contact with parents. This socially sanctioned behavior can be emotionally crippling, for separating from parents is an important aspect of our distinguishing ourselves as full adults—but comes with no guarantee that we will feel mature.

Cheryl came to therapy because of chronic depression and low self-esteem. She made few independent decisions; she consulted her mother about raising her children, what to buy, even what to cook for dinner. At forty, Cheryl feels incompetent and sees herself as another child among her own children because she cannot separate from her mother. Our therapy focused on Cheryl taking independent steps and making independent choices apart from me or her mother in order to build her self-esteem.

Flight: To avoid the confrontation of the grief of separating, many of us simply flee. Most common is when a date, acquaintance, or lover never calls again rather than address any uncomfortable feelings in the relationship. Several unhappily married women told me of their secret fantasy of leaving their husbands silently in the middle of the night to avoid confrontation or the pain of parting. Occasionally people do separate in this devastating way, leaving a partner or family bereft and helpless.

The first time he took a separate vacation from his parents, Rod never returned again. Alive and well 3,000 miles from his family, this young man saw no way out of his family except to secretly flee. The same is true of Sam, a young husband who never returned to his wife and child after a camping trip. Although no body was found, he was presumed dead, only to turn up years later alive in another city, in another life. A great inability to communicate or cope with feelings causes one to flee, and yet these flights out of relationships create enormous pain for the people involved.

Thoughts of dying: When we feel powerless, we may want to die. Not only does the idea of separating set off our primitive fears of dying if we part, but sometimes we also find separating so difficult to face that we consider dying instead of separating and living on. Occasionally people do commit suicide rather than live through the experience of someone leaving them or a relationship ending. Fortunately, few of us act on these thoughts, even though many of us have thoughts of dying in response to the loss of a loved one. When we have suicidal thoughts, we are out of touch with our courage and our ability to renew ourselves and regenerate our lives. We may need others' help to recover ourselves. The more natural path, whether we like it or not, is to grow from adversity, not to die from it.

Anger: A common and indirect means we use to leave one another is through anger. For the majority of us, anger, more than any other reason, justifies saying good-bye and letting go. Anger mobilizes us to act. Anger masks our sorrow or regret and makes us feel strong and powerful. Young people often angrily free themselves from parents in order to be independent. For lots of us anger is essential for accomplishing a separation from either parents, children, spouses, friends, or jobs.

A client, Cindy, told me the only way she could leave her husband was to keep herself at a high enough pitch of anger and resentment to bolster her through the process of separating. She was afraid that if she let her angry feelings go, she might soften toward her husband and not have the strength or feel she had the right to leave her unhappy marriage.

When mutual trust breaks down, couples may become mired in anger. I have known many couples who were simply hateful to each other in order to separate—free of sorrow, loneliness, guilt, or regret. We may rage our way out of our relationships to deny the depths of our fears. Some of us couldn't leave under any other circumstances, or we could not stay apart if we didn't stay angry.

Criticism: Another common way we separate is to criticize and devalue the other person, to crush love out in advance of separating in order to avoid any sorrow or regret. Grown children often devalue their parents in order to leave home. A common maneuver, especially used by immature and young people, is to make love unimaginable or the other person unimportant, unreal, or valueless to counter any sense of loss or sadness. Little children push away by saying, "I didn't love you anyway." As adults, we pick apart our partner in detail as a preliminary to and a justification for ending an unhappy relationship. We may succeed in separating that way, but we also unnecessarily hurt, undermine, or damage our partner at the same time. We also undermine ourselves, for then we wonder, "What kind of a jerk was I to love him?"

Blame: Because of our tendency to make ourselves right and others wrong, we self-righteously blame the other person and see ourselves as blameless for whatever problems exist between us. That way we can look good and be free of guilt or responsibility for the relationship having failed. Like criticizing, blaming our partner allows us to bolster ourselves and justify our leaving. Blaming, we avoid taking responsibility for or learning about what makes relationships work. Unaware of ourselves, we are apt to repeat the same scenario with subsequent partners.

FORCING RELATIONSHIPS TO CONTINUE: BY FEAR OR MANIPULATION

Fear: Although many fears are associated with separation, a crippling fear is that if we leave something terrible will happen to ourselves or the other person. The worst fantasy is that one of us will die. Probably three-quarters of my clients who want to separate or divorce express fear that their partner would

133

somehow die or commit suicide if left. This common fear usually has little basis in reality, but we manipulate ourselves into staying in relationships because of it.

Such fear is stimulated by our faulty belief that our own or another's survival depends on our relationship, which may be projections of our own neediness, our own survival feelings or fears. Many of us have been afraid that we would die if left, or we remember wanting to die when a relationship ended. These are not unusual thoughts, but thinking about giving up and dying is very different from our actually doing so. Typically, partners who are left not only survive but also create better lives for themselves, although a few will resist generating meaningful new lives.

Manipulation: Some of us will do anything, manipulate in any way we can, to avoid the pain of separation. To fight for a relationship to continue is not unhealthy, but dirty fighting is. One partner may attempt to cajole or overpower the other into staying in a relationship by threats to their person, or to whatever they hold dear, such as children, family, home, or money. Threatening to die is the most extreme manipulation, a powerful form of emotional blackmail employed by a desperate, immature person. Most of us are afraid to risk challenging these kinds of manipulations, and we may need to get professional help to do so.

SEPARATING SUCCESSFULLY

We have had many examples of how indirect we are in dealing with separation, avoiding the natural feelings inherent in parting. Each of us needs to be able to separate and still feel whole and satisfied with ourselves and those from whom we part.

Facing the issues, communicating about them, and not having to be "right" all help us successfully separate.

Facing the issues: The truth is usually easier to face than we imagine it will be, if we will look at it squarely. Our avoidance is what makes things so difficult. Because another wants to leave a relationship doesn't mean that we are bad or inadequate or unlovable, any more than our wish to leave makes them or us bad or wrong. As discussed earlier, we all change our hearts and minds at times and will want to end a relationship. That's uncomfortable but also human, and we can learn to cope with it.

Owning and communicating feelings: Healthy separating involves noticing, allowing, and acknowledging our feelings fully and being direct and honest with others. This means expressing ourselves and listening to the other person's feelings and attitudes as well. At this time especially we would be wise not to personalize or dramatize feelings. Open communication lies at the heart of successful parting and successful relating. Openly sharing ourselves enables us to part more amicably and to feel better about ourselves and the other person as well. When we deal directly with our relationship issues and with our feelings about leaving or being left, both parties can grow and mature.

Many of us envision that if we shared our true feelings we would feel too guilty to leave. We may worry that we would never leave if we had loving feelings toward the other person. This is a difficult truth to grasp: We can love someone with whom we do not wish to continue sharing our lives. Loving another and wanting to be with that person are not the same thing. However, the best means for knowing how we really feel is through communicating, not by imagining how we feel.

Not having to be "right": So often we would rather be right than resolve issues. Self-righteousness inhibits communication and resolution. We could separate and complete our relationships in more satisfying ways if we gave up having to be right. Ideally, we could sit down together and share our appreciations, resentments, joys, sorrows, regrets, hopes, and disappointments. We could both fully allow and express our feelings and hear those of our partner. Then we could accept and forgive ourselves and each other. "Good-bye" could be an opening for each of us to move forward in life. Although "good-bye" might still hurt, it need not be devastating.

My friends Franny and Ernest sought therapy to complete their ten-year marriage amicably so that they could continue to successfully co-parent without having to go on living together. In three sessions, they expressed their resentments and appreciations for one another until they reached a point where they felt able to just be friends without hurt or anger or blame. They acknowledged their disappointment at ending their marriage, and they accepted their choice to separate not as a failure but as a change. These two people have inspired me and many others, for they accomplished the rare feat of ending their marriage successfully. They did not have a painless ending, since endings are not necessarily painless, but they had a fully expressed and complete ending.

Another couple who tried this same means to end their relationship cleared up so many issues in the process that instead of parting they made new marriage vows. Communication is our most powerful tool toward resolution. (For more about completion and forgiveness, see chapters 22 and 23.)

• 19 •

OVERCOMING GRIEF

Grief is the agony of an instant;
the indulgence of grief the blunder of a life.
BENJAMIN DISRAELI, *VIRGINIA GREY*

Of all the experiences we ever confront in life, the loss of
people we love is by far the most painful and often the
hardest from which to recover. Our most intense emotional
experiences and our greatest suffering are usually associated
with loss and grief, and we are most apt to become bogged down
and stay unresolved with our feelings of loss. For most of us it is
intolerable to say good-bye. In *The Courage to Grieve* I wrote that it
takes courage to grieve, and yet equally important is the courage
it takes to let go of grief.

Because we don't know how to grieve and how to let grief
go, we sometimes do horrible things to ourselves in response
to grief. So many examples come to mind, like the thirty-five-
year-old mother of two who denied herself any personal life
as she grieved for thirteen years after her young husband died
of cancer. As a result of our brief therapy together, she finally
let herself resume living, began socializing, and, symbolically,
bought herself a new red car. Another woman told me she read

her dead mother's letters and cried every day for twenty-seven years. I met a sixty-year-old woman whose body had rigidified and demeanor changed to that of an eighty-year-old after her husband's sudden death. I talked to the family of a man who had not stopped raging for the three years since his son died in an accident. He had so alienated his boss that he lost his job, and so frightened his wife and other children that they dared not speak to him. I received a letter from a young English girl who went to bed for three years when her boyfriend left her, and another from an older British woman consumed with bitterness and hate because her family died before her. I have met many people frozen with sorrow, rage, and guilt over loved ones' suicides. These are just a few of the many disturbing examples of people who nearly destroyed their lives with grief.

It seems to me that the best testimonial we can give to our dead loved ones is how well we recover and live our lives after a loss, not how much we grieve. Our misconception is in imagining that our suffering or how intensely or how long we grieve is a measure of how much we loved. In truth, none of us would want another's grief as a testimonial of their love for us. More likely we would want our loved ones to live healthy, fulfilled lives without us.

Although grieving is inevitable, recovering from grief is not. Thus, my concern has been, "How can we recover ourselves and be complete with our pain more quickly and more easily?" Since writing *The Courage to Grieve,* I have discovered that we have more choice about how, how much, and how long we grieve. The current belief is that the onslaught to the psyche due to loss is so overwhelming that it necessarily takes many months to recover and that we must live through every symbolic event or anniversary in order to let go. Now it is evident to me that we can have more choice and more freedom than that.

This is not to deny how painful and disturbing grief can be, for grief can be overwhelming and bewildering. Grief can feel like "craziness," and the complexity and intensity of it can be very frightening, particularly for those of us who need to maintain control of ourselves. However, even though we may experience strong emotions when we grieve, we do not have to stay overwhelmed. The important distinction here is: Do we have emotions or do our emotions have us?

THE NATURAL EXPERIENCE OF GRIEF

Grief is a natural and healthy response to loss, disappointment, and change. We grieve over changes in our bodies, illnesses, accidents, or any hardships or traumatic events in our lives, and we grieve as we grow and discover new aspects of ourselves. We may grieve for who we once were, or for how our lives have been. Most of us associate grief with the loss of loved ones, whether through death, separation, or divorce. Loss is fraught with anguish for most of us. We may weep, feeling sadness, regret, anger, and other emotions. Unfortunately, many of us don't know what healthy grief is or how to grieve.

As natural as it is, the expressing of our grief is something we often suppress. We do not allow ourselves to cry, and we deny our sadness or any uncomfortable feelings. We are afraid to let the floodgates open, afraid to open our hearts fully to our pain, lest we be overwhelmed or never recover. Our desire to appear "grown-up" or controlled stops us from allowing ourselves to feel deeply, and so we hold our grief in and never let it go, never complete it. Our unexpressed griefs simply persist through time, influencing our relationships and our actions. Because our suppressed emotions cause a lot of tension in our everyday lives, I have taken to suggesting to people that the bottom line on dissolving grief is this: Never miss an opportunity to cry.

HOW WE PERPETUATE THE SUFFERING OF GRIEF

Traditionally, how we grieve is debilitating. If we don't suppress or deny our grief, we overextend it. Because we hold the loss of our loved ones to be pitiful and traumatic, we intensify and prolong our suffering. We get stuck in the grief process in only partially experiencing our feelings, or in not letting go of our feelings, thoughts, or memories. We also turn our upsetting feelings into obsessive preoccupations.

Often we are unaware that we intensify our own pain. (See part II.) We add to our suffering and cause it to last indefinitely by embracing and glorifying our feelings, by constantly reminding ourselves of our loss and our memories, by extending our feelings over time, and by our distorted ideas about loss and death. Unfortunately, many of us get "stuck" in living the story of our loss every day, for our identity or idea of ourselves becomes that of someone who has suffered a loss. We intensify our pain by immersing ourselves in memories, romanticizing our memories, and being sentimental. Today's love songs bear this out. We do not need to erase our memories, but putting our memories, photographs, or mementos away for now may be instrumental in helping us to heal.

More than anything else, our beliefs keep us in pain and hold us back from full recovery. The idea that our relationships should last forever causes us the most anguish. Our grief is often immense because we are so unprepared when relationships end or people die. Although we can choose to love people forever, we cannot guarantee another person's presence in our lives forever or for any period of time. Nothing, absolutely nothing, lasts forever, yet somehow we are always surprised by "endings." We cannot seem to tolerate the transience of nature, of human life, and of our connections with one another.

Many of us are compelled to grieve long after a loss has occurred. We may continue grieving to express our love, as if letting go of our sorrow would invalidate our love or our relationship. By grieving to perpetuate the "specialness" of our love, we stay mired in endless grieving instead of living. Sometimes we maintain grief to punish the one who left us or someone else, or because we fear being alone, or change, or the unknown. Either way, the tragic result is that we maintain relationships with dead people instead of living people.

Another limiting belief is that grief lasts forever, which we prove by never letting go. Many times we hold our own loss or circumstance to be so unique that we see ourselves as the exception to any possible recovery, especially if we lose people under terrible or shocking circumstances. However, no matter what our circumstances, we can recover and go on with living. This was made obvious to me in a grief workshop I led by a couple whose twenty-two-year-old daughter was murdered by her boyfriend. Theirs was such a traumatic and dramatic loss that the other workshop participants were riveted to whatever these two people had to say. They shared their realization that their only choice was to go on living, and so they recovered even from this tragic event.

The idea that we are victims of a loss perpetuates our grief. It is natural to feel like victims when someone suddenly disappears from our lives, and we may feel like victims because of the onslaught of the varying and intense emotions that grief can entail. We may feel singled out because we feel pain or because of the circumstances of our loss or trauma. Other people's pity or solace can add to our feeling victimized.

However, seeing ourselves as victims weakens us and impedes our healing and recovering. Once we feel victimized, we feel powerless. We need to remember that we do not necessarily have to be victims of our emotions, that how we grieve and how long we grieve can be our choice. Nor do we have to feel like victims of our circumstances, whatever they may be. But to overcome feeling victimized, we need to be willing to recover, willing to be open to life anew.

Even though we may not be aware of it, we always have a choice: Grief can be a brief moment or a many months' break in our living. I now suspect that our commonly held belief/tradition of a year or two for mourning may give us permission to live too long amidst debilitating emotions. It is radical and also exciting to realize that in fact grief can actually be complete in days or weeks. The speed with which we finish with grief is totally dependent on whether we are committed to completion or to suffering.

COMPLETING OR FINISHING WITH GRIEF

What does finishing with grief entail? Completion is literally saying "good-bye" to the one we have lost and letting go of all the emotions, all the anguish surrounding the loss itself. Completion of grief is not ending our love, forgetting our loved one, or erasing our memories, but it is the releasing of ourselves from pain.

Moving our grief from the foreground of our lives into the background is the most critical step toward healing from a loss. To be truly complete, we must be willing to detach ourselves from both the one we lost and from our grief. This means disengaging ourselves from having grief be the most important aspect of our lives and from having the one we lost be the only important person to us, even when the one we lost has been our closest person. Although difficult, this is what will give us the most relief and will allow us to begin our lives anew.

The willingness to be complete with grief is a stand we take, rather than a natural outcome. The idea of completion seems no more natural to us than grieving itself, even though both are natural. Too many of us are walking around in pain today from past losses, grieving as a habit. Therefore, first we have to be willing to stop grieving. Then, as paradoxical as it may seem, to complete grief we need to experience it, to allow and express *all* of our related feelings—sadness, anger, or whatever. Expressing feelings allows them to disappear. Then, after we have allowed our feelings, we need to be willing to stop torturing ourselves. The method for completing grief is described in detail in the subsequent chapter on Completion.

Finally, we need to examine our commitment: Is it to suffering or to not suffering? If we are now committed to not suffering, then to support our decision to let go we may need to set a specific date in time by which we intend to be finished grieving. We can promise ourselves that our grief will be over in one week or in one month. We can, if we are willing and committed to do so, live out that promise by consciously behaving in ways that we know would support our healing (See part IV.)

We will need support to keep our promise not to suffer any further. Most important, we must let go of any interfering beliefs or behaviors. We cannot indulge in nostalgia or "reruns" of our history of the circumstances of our loss or perpetuate self-pity, anger, bitterness, or hopelessness. Remember, our biggest fight to heal may be in resisting our own thoughts. We must be willing to take charge of ourselves, our lives, and our future and be willing to reach out for whatever support from other people we need to keep us on the track of healing ourselves instead of staying mired in grief. People can be a great help at this time. We can ask others to remind us of our promise to heal or to listen, to check in on us, or to join us in some enlivening activity. We can also engage in projects or activities that involve us in living instead of grieving to help us keep our promise not to suffer anymore.

We can discover if we are more committed to suffering than we are to recovering by looking at our behaviors. If we don't keep our word, and we keep moving back into our pain, chances are we may be more committed than we realized to grieving. We are apt to grieve extensively when we commit to a lengthy or sentimental testimonial to our lost or dead loved one. An example of this is how at seventeen, after my brother died, I promised myself to think of him every day of my life. It is no surprise that my grief lasted for many years. I would never weigh myself down with such a promise today. In contrast, when we are committed to have our grief end, we let go of our pain more quickly and effortlessly.

For the future, being complete in our relationships is the single most important action we can take to enable us to deal with loss. Being up-to-date with all the communications and actions we wish to take with loved ones, having no loose ends, is a powerful tool for being able to let go quickly and easily. Being complete is a good habit that we can initiate immediately.

ACCEPTING DEATH AS NATURAL

Our ideas about death have a major impact on how we survive losses. People's responses to my parents' deaths showed

144

me that. Instead of simply accepting the end of life as inevitable, we invariably perceive the end of our time here as tragic, unexpected, and absolute. My brother's sudden death was traumatic, for at seventeen I had no context for death except as an absolute ending. I can see now how much having a specific context in which we hold death helps us cope with loss. It was many years before I understood the message in my recurrent dreams about my brother, who told me over and over that he lived someplace else, a place without telephones or addresses. Years later I realized he was telling me of his life after death.

The realization that our soul or spirit is eternal has given me enormous solace, even in the times when I have missed terribly those I have lost. We can always know our dead loved ones are with us in spirit. Our losses then do not have to seem quite so tragic as when we think of death as absolute. For me, death is sometimes like having a long-distance relationship with a friend or loved one whom I love but never see. For those of us who need more evidence or information about this, I recommend reading Kenneth Ring's *Life as Death, An Investigation of Near Death Experiences,* and Reverend Raymond A. Moody's *Life After Life.*

We can choose how we perceive death, even allowing that death is inevitable. Even though we may not know for sure what happens after our bodies die, why not just trust the age-old messages that our souls are eternal? Is there any better alternative? By doing so, we would eliminate so much of the fear and drama and misery we add to our good-byes with loved ones, as well as make easier our confrontation with our own inevitable demise. Accepting that our souls are everlasting may free us of much of our suffering in confronting the deaths of those we love. We may also free the dead to go on more easily to whatever is next for them.

I began writing this book a few weeks after my father's death to express my commitment to going on with my life, to let my father know I would make it without him, and to say that each of us can transcend our grief. It is not from lack of tears, pain, or suffering that I came to these conclusions. Quite the opposite. I cried a great deal before my father died. My family used to call me the girl who "wore her heart on her sleeve," but when I lost my parents, I chose not to do so. The important message here is that grief and loss are unavoidable, and yet how we grieve and how long we suffer is truly our choice, no matter what our circumstances are. All of this discussion is meant to free us to make such choices for ourselves.

•20•

Our Relationship with Our Parents

Children begin by loving their parents;
after a time they judge them;
rarely, if ever, do they forgive them.

Oscar Wilde

Our relationship with our parents, whether they are alive or dead, is often a lifelong area of conflict and distress. Even if they are not in our lives, their spirit, their impact, is with us forever. They are the source of our lives, yet few of us experience gratitude or appreciate that. Instead, for many of us our relationship with our parents is a source of suffering.

Since we universally expect parents to be perfect, we are invariably disappointed when our parents err. All parents make mistakes, and yet we treat parents' errors as criminal acts against us. We don't seem to realize that our parents are simply human and so bound to have problems, peculiarities, and limitations. In being unwilling to accept our parents' fallibility, some of us continue maligning our parents forever. Others of us closed the book on our parents long ago because of the injuries we imagine they inflicted on us.

WE BLAME OUR PARENTS

While other cultures revere parents, in our culture we blame parents for what we consider the damage they have done to us. Even if we do not see them as damaging us, we view our parents at least as a stumbling block and the probable cause of our difficulties later in life. When we do acknowledge their influence on our lives, we often see only their negative impact on us, in our personal characteristics, problems, limitations, and dissatisfactions. We malign our parents, and we hold them responsible for everything they ever said or did, even years later. We use our parents to justify our difficulties in life or in other relationships, our lack of satisfaction, or our failure to achieve our goals. Parents make perfect scapegoats since they invariably make mistakes. Because we never forget, we stay bogged down in our relationship with our parents.

Blaming our parents as we do is another way we hold ourselves to be victims in life. We diminish our power this way, and we never fully grow up. Each of us needs to come to terms with our parents, alive or dead, regardless of how they treated us, so that we can be full-fledged adults ourselves. We need to release them and forgive them their mistakes in order to free ourselves. To be complete with our parents, we need to realize that most parents do the very best they can at any moment, no matter how it looked to us. (There are exceptions—disturbed and cruel people—who do not fit in this discussion, yet we need to be complete with them nonetheless.)

WE EXPECT TOO MUCH OF OUR PARENTS

Our impossible expectations are the cause of much of our misery with our parents. We expect parents to be fully grown-up, to know the right thing to do, to be wise, and to behave impeccably at all times. Even more, we expect our parents to be free of problems. We want to be raised by superhumans instead of humans.

Our primary mistake in regard to our parents is that we imagine that they should have known better. How could they? Clearly, being a parent does not guarantee being grown-up. They arrived at the job of parent untrained and likely unskilled; possibly it was a job thrust upon them rather than a job they sought. They learned to parent by either automatically avoiding or copying the example set by their own parents, or else experimenting, which tends to be hit or miss.

Even with extensive birth control and so many births by choice, we forget that our parents did not necessarily choose to be parents. Often they became pregnant and then dealt with parenthood. All at once they had to recover from the shock of our impending arrival and learn how to parent. For some, this adjustment to parenting must have been like suddenly and unexpectedly having to learn to fly an airplane—not easy. On top of it all, being a parent is a full-time, twenty-four-hour-a-day job that may last eighteen years or more. Once they took on the job, they had to start from scratch to raise us, support us, and live with us every day for many years to come. Being a parent is an enormous commitment.

Another difficulty implicit in parenting is that children often resist and react to changes and separations of even short duration by feeling abandoned or unloved. Children may react strongly when breast-feeding ends, or bottles are taken away, or when parents leave to go out to work or to socialize, or when other siblings are born. Any of these natural events can be a trauma for which we blame our parents—sometimes forever.

It is not unusual for us to feel fear or anger or pain or rejection when separated from our parents. Unfortunately, some of us never let go of our reactions to these early natural separations. As a psychotherapist, I see how often as adults we persist in blaming our parents for the birth of a sibling or for being sent to kindergarten or for having to stay with a baby-sitter. Even years later, we seem particularly sensitive to any proof that our parents abandoned us. We persist in viewing our experiences from the same vantage point as long ago, and we forget the past is over. We do not realize that we can be complete now with *any* event from the past. (See chapter 23: Completing Our Experiences.)

CONSEQUENCES OF BLAME AND EXPECTATIONS

Blaming our parents for our problems in life has grim consequences. When we shut our parents out of our lives, we lose their love and support and we cut off or deny a piece of ourselves. Then we view ourselves as deprived or damaged, an outlook that subsequently influences every aspect of our lives. Equally tragic is that we doom ourselves to forever feeling victimized and therefore powerless.

The fact of blaming in itself, rather than the wrongs our parents supposedly committed, can be the cause of many of our difficulties later in life. For instance, blaming our father can begin a pattern of blaming all men, or all people in authority, or all people. Unforgiving, our energies are simply tied up elsewhere. Unfortunately, the chances are that if we are still blaming our parents, we are limited in our ability to love anyone else.

ABUSIVE PARENTS

Some parents do terrible damage to their children in the forms of physical, sexual, or verbal abuse. Abusive parents are often immature, psychologically troubled, and damaged people themselves who need a great deal of help. Unfortunately, people are not selected for parenthood on the basis of their maturity or ability.

We can recover from abusive parenting. We may need help to do so—either psychotherapeutic help or the help of support groups, like Adult Children of Alcoholics. However, people are amazingly resilient. Over the years I have seen terrible pain inflicted on people by their parents, and yet these same people live useful and healthy lives. Bill was severely beaten as a child, and still he became a wise, loving, and able adult, in part because a loving grandmother softened the blows. This man does not beat his wife or children. Instead, he is a popular coach of Little League and a favored boss. Jimmy, dragged from city to city by an alcoholic mother, was exposed to hunger, filth, brutality, and his mother's frequent sexual encounters. Jimmy is a loving, bright, and fun husband, father, and friend. I met him socially, not as a client, and was amazed that this marvelous man had survived so much trauma as a child.

Years ago without warning my best friend's mother walked out on her husband and three young children. I could not imagine that my ten-year-old friend, Sally, could recover from this inexplicable trauma. Yet Sally turned to her friends for support and went on to be a class leader. Today she is a happy and successful mother, wife, and career woman. We can survive, recover, and succeed even after traumatic events in our childhoods.

HEALING OUR RELATIONSHIPS WITH OUR PARENTS

We each must come to terms with our relationship with our parents. All of us have suffered in some way from our parents, although not necessarily as painfully as in the examples above. Grief seems to be implicit in being a child and in being a parent. We grieve over what happened or what never happened. We cannot erase what was, but we can take the "sting" out or our emphasis off it. We also grieve over parting from each other, whether we are just leaving home or our parents die.

We can take charge of our experiences from the past by facing them and owning them, instead of being victims of them. They are over. We can further take charge of our past by accepting that it is too late now to fill in the gaps, that we cannot get what we never got from our parents, be it mother love or nurturing or financial support or whatever yearnings we bring forward from our childhood. Those days and those possibilities are over. We need to accept and forgive what did or did not happen. My experience is that the people who "hang on" to unsatisfying relationships with their parents as adults are those who have felt the most deprived. Those of us who have gotten the least from our parents are most apt to stay around much too long trying to get what we never got.

The most important thing for us as adults to do about our childhood is to consciously and willingly let it go. Then we can be full adults. Then we can be free to live and love and be fully present and open to our lives. Too, we have the possibility of having a more equal and satisfying relationship with our parents, if they are around.

We must forgive our parents if we can, no matter how terrible the wrongs done to us. It's in our own best interest to disengage ourselves from blaming our parents any longer. In *The Prince of Tides,* Pat Conroy made this point: "My life did not really begin until I summoned the power to forgive my father for making my childhood a long march of terror." Without forgiveness we are handicapped and constricted, stuck in the past, filled with hurt or resentment that prevents us from fully trusting and fully living, from loving and being loved. Unforgiving, we get to live halfheartedly, at best.

Acknowledging that our parents loved us is the first step to forgiving them, even though we may have had objections or questions about the form of our parents' love. Whatever their style of lovingness, we need to admit their love. This can be the end of our griping, complaining, and justifying our misery, limitations, or problems. And if they were actually too disturbed to love, we need to forgive them their lack, their limitations, in order to free ourselves from them. Chances are they committed years of their lives to our welfare and survival. If they are alive today, most likely they are still committed to our welfare, no matter how it looks to us. Acknowledge them for what they gave. Acknowledging our parents is a critical step in our taking responsibility for our own lives and in expanding our ability to relate to other people.

We need to see our parents newly. Many of us stay "stuck" with our parents by seeing them only as our parents instead of as the people they are in the world. To regain our power over our lives we must start fresh and relate to our parents as they are now, as people, as friends, as other adults. This means completing with our parents as our parents, accepting them as people. We need to forgive them so that we can allow them to step out of the role of parent into the experience of being a person for us.

One way to complete our past with them is to express appreciations as much as resentments or regrets. We might acknowledge past difficulties or simply let them know we love them. We can let them know what they most want to know, which is that they got their job done with us, that we are fine.

THE GESTALT THERAPY TECHNIQUE FOR LETTING GO

Regardless of whether our parents are now living or dead, available or not, we each need to have some means of letting go of the story of our past—the memories, the incidents, the hurts, and the disappointments. We do not need to tell our parents every gripe or disappointment in order to be complete, since that could pointlessly reopen old wounds. We do need to allow the past to be released and forgiven and forgotten. We gain our power over our past more by declaring ourselves finished with our parents and our childhood once and for all than by retelling the story.

Having an imaginary conversation *aloud* with each parent can be an effective way to complete with parents, alive or dead. Empty chairs or pillows or photographs can represent our parents' places in this dialogue. Use this opportunity to express *all* of your unfinished business, your disappointments, hurts, regrets, and recriminations, with the intention of emptying out the past, saying good-bye to it, and being complete forever. Rather than putting your parents through all of your historical feelings, this kind of forgiving is best done on your private time rather than directly with your parents.

FORGIVING OUR PARENTS

I cannot say this strongly enough: It is critical to forgive our parents as a way to free ourselves to have full and satisfying lives today. I know there are terrible parents, but whatever they did to us is now over; we need to live in the present. Some of us will not stop blaming and will not forgive. Even though we may be fearful of taking charge of our life or are more comfortable being run by past, familiar circumstances, we can generate much more satisfying lives today by letting all the past incidents go. (See part IV, chapters 22 and 23.)

Once we approach our parents from an attitude of forgiveness, we may see them very differently than before and appreciate them from a totally new perspective. We may see their criticisms as loving. Their demands or harshness may reflect how responsible they felt as our parents, or their leniency may represent their faith in us.

As an adult, Ted developed a new perspective on his father. Ted's father, a Marine Corps officer, instructed Ted to rake the stones and rocks surrounding their desert home daily after school as a teenager. Ted thought his father was "crazy" then, but years later Ted sees that his father taught him commitment, impeccability, and perseverance.

As a child, Tom blamed his parents that he was born handicapped with cerebral palsy. As an adult, Tom took on chairmanship of the Holiday Project, which involves visiting institutionalized people at holiday times, out of his special empathy for these people and to express his deep gratitude to his parents that he did not have to spend his life in an institution. Like Ted, Tom can now acknowledge his parents. Perhaps the best gift we can give our parents is our realization and acknowledgment of and gratitude for the fact that they are the source of who we are in the world.

VIEWING OUR PARENTS FROM A NEW PERSPECTIVE

We might alter our whole view of our lives if we experimented with the idea that we chose our parents. This perspective gives us some power over our lives and eliminates the idea that we are victims of fate. The idea that these two people are exactly who we intended to have raise us can release us from our judgments, disappointments, and grievances.

In examining why we would choose these exact two people to be our parents, we might see what special lessons or advantages were available to us out of this particular choice. We may see that, in choosing a parent who was a harsh taskmaster, we learned discipline and commitment. For me, choosing a father who was a busy doctor initiated me into service-type work. Choosing a devoted mother may have enabled us to have the confidence to take on big jobs in life or to love others, while choosing a cold mother may have taught us necessary independence. There are always lessons in our relationships with our parents, whether we see them or not, and in reflecting this way we could be responsible for choosing to learn them.

We might also imagine our parents chose us to be their children, another way to get an overview of our lives that may modify our complaints about the form of our parents' love. This will also cut out the stories that we didn't please our parents, that we were meant to be a different sex or a different kind of person. Considering ourselves chosen, we'd know that our parents loved and wanted us, no matter how they behaved. How much better we would feel about ourselves and our parents to think, "My parents wanted a rough and tumble little boy," or "My parents wanted a shy little girl," or "I was the wanted sixth child."

Another possibility is that we can choose new parents if we cannot relate to our own parents. Parents can and do fail. Sometimes, no matter how or what we do, we cannot fully resolve our relationship with them. They may be estranged from us, or mentally or physically ill. Instead of beating our heads against the same old walls, trying to get what is not there for us, we need to let go of our expectations and perhaps look elsewhere.

At any age or under any circumstances, we can ask other adults, if they are willing, to serve in the role of our mother or father. We can seek a new parent to help us temporarily get through a crisis or for long-term intimacy. We can then pick exactly what we want for ourselves now. We can expand our lives at any time by choosing new parents or siblings or children to receive and give the love we may be missing.

When I shared this idea in a workshop years ago, sixteen-year-old Michael asked me to be his mother. I was delighted to be chosen. For several years, until he moved away, we maintained a mutually rewarding, loving relationship, which far surpassed either of our ideas of a good parent-child relationship.

MAKE YOURSELF HAPPY NOW

As conscious adults, we can create a life for ourselves now that fills in the gaps of what we missed. Just as we can choose new parents, we can choose new children or any new family. We can buy ourselves the train our parents would never buy us, or indulge in candy, or stay up all night, or do whatever we missed doing. As children, we thought it was our parents' job to make us happy. Now we know that is not true. No one can make us happy but us. So let's make ourselves happy! You can give yourself a happy childhood today.

We can stop having our relationships with our parents be a source of suffering and instead appreciate our parents as the source of our lives—if we will only forgive them and begin fresh with them today. To come to terms with our parents, we need to admit, accept, and allow them to be as they are. We need to let the past be over for us, to grieve if we need to grieve, and to forgive them and ourselves. This will free us to function independently and successfully in our own lives and perhaps to have a new richness in our relationship with our parents. As Anna told her five-year-old daughter, "Please don't just remember me for my mistakes."

• 21 •

Our Bodies and Our Health

*We are, in real life, a reasonably healthy people. Far from being
ineptly put together, we are amazingly tough, durable organisms,
full of health, ready for most contingencies."*

Lewis Thomas, *The Medusa and the Snail*

Our bodies and our health problems are often a source of
suffering. Any ill health can be a traumatic event or a cri
sis in our lives. At the same time, our health problems can be
a reaction to the stresses or difficulties in our lives. Sometimes
we may cope with or resolve problems with symptoms and disease as well. Since physical symptoms serve these three contrast-
ing functions, it is not surprising that the whole area of physical
health and illness tends to be complicated and mysterious for
most of us.

We often have a poor relationship with our bodies, akin to
relating to a being from another planet, since our bodies can
seem totally foreign to us. We are bewildered by how our bodies
work or respond, and we become frightened when our bodies
do not work well. We often treat our bodies the way we treat
our automobiles, hoping they will get us through life, hoping

they will not break down, but not doing much to understand them or maintain them in good working order. Some of us take better care of our cars than our bodies.

We think we have no power over our health because we do not understand how our bodies work. We imagine that health, like good luck, is bestowed by fate or the "powers that be" rather than being self-generated. Thus, any kind of physical change or problem can trigger our "victim consciousness." Any ill health, even a minor medical problem like a wart, a muscle ache, or a cold, can set off a cycle of anxiety and worry. And if we contract something more serious like pneumonia or cancer, we are apt to be immobilized.

There is a natural interaction and interrelationship between the mind and body; this is the most important thing for us to know about our bodies. When we feel pressed or over-whelmed by our emotions or our circumstances, our body can be stressed in such a way as to produce physical symptoms. Upset, we may develop a headache, a sore throat, diarrhea, or an inexplicable pain. When we don't express our feelings, they may show up in our body as pains or infections. Because our bodies are always influenced by our minds, much illness is "psychosomatic." However, we usually use the word "psycho-somatic" to judge or blame ourselves for causing symptoms, instead of using this concept as a new, valuable tool for improving our health.

PHYSICAL PROBLEMS SERVE MANY PURPOSES

Physical symptoms may serve any of several functions, all of which are meant to assist us, not hurt us. Although they may appear as the "enemy" sometimes, our bodies are an integral part of us and a support. Symptoms can reflect problems, alert us to difficulties or deeper feelings, express feelings that we have withheld or suppressed, be a reaction to problems, or protect us from something that we have trouble facing. Once we have looked at each of these functions, we will look at ways to reveal or discover what a symptom is saying.

We are often unaware of how much our bodies reflect our inner truths. Jim Simkin, who trained me in Gestalt therapy, often said, "Our bodies never lie." Our true feelings are revealed through our physical being, if not expressed directly through words. All of us have experienced times when our physical symptoms reflected unexpressed or unresolved problems, emotions or reactions. When we denied ourselves the freedom to weep, we developed a runny nose or a cold. We have felt body pains or generated a rash when we suppressed anger. Sometimes our frustrations have turned into a throbbing headache or stomach cramps. Facing very stressful events like the severe illnesses and hospitalizations of family members and friends, I noticed I hurt all over. It is not unusual to develop an uncomfortable symptom or a full-blown illness in response to a specific painful incident, some suppressed emotion, or general stress.

Physical symptoms often serve to alert us to hidden difficulties, signaling us that something is wrong. We may notice a physical reaction before we know we are having an emotional upheaval. A headache or a cold may trigger our noticing some unhappiness or conflict. Persistent symptoms, like headaches, backaches, upset stomachs, diarrhea, or chronic colds, can be the impetus for looking more deeply at our lives or for seeking help. These "wake-up calls" from our body are often so glaring and unavoidable that they move us to act. Once we begin to express our upsetting feelings or to deal with the problem or to alter our lives to resolve our situation, the symptom diminishes or disappears.

Many of us get sick when confronted with adversity. We don't always develop physical symptoms after stressful experiences, but we can. Our bodies react to loss or threatened separation, to conflict, hardship, trauma, and sudden life changes. We may develop symptoms in response to any upsetting or stressful emotional experience or any internal conflict that involves strong feelings like guilt, shame, regret, ambivalence, or hurt. Sometimes we get sick when we try to resist or avoid something in our lives. More is being learned all the time about this phenomenon of becoming ill in reaction to experiences that are unexpressed and unresolved. Carl Simonton and Stephanie Matthews-Simonton have been pioneers in this work with emotional factors with cancer patients, and they have co-authored (with James Creighton) a very helpful book sharing their wisdom called *Getting Well Again* (J. P. Tarcher, 1978). Another brilliant book on this subject is *Love, Medicine and Miracles* by Bernie Siegel (Harper & Row, 1986).

Our body functions to serve us, although it may not always appear so. We may develop a symptom to protect us from taking a step that is distressful to our inner being. Clients have become ill before an inadvisable marriage or an unwanted vacation or when too much is expected of them. I became incapacitated just before a trip to climb a mountain, later realizing that my fear of injury led me to become ill instead of going.

We may become sick in order to stop or rest or regroup or be taken care of. When we are not aware enough to tell ourselves to act or slow down or to reconsider a plan or to stop, our bodies may indicate those needs through physical symptoms or illness.

We may use illness to retreat from our problems, to literally hide under the covers. Like drugs, illness can numb us to difficulties in our lives since we can become so preoccupied with our physical complaints that we barely remember the stress that provoked us to be ill. Lots of us use disease and ill health to avoid confronting life. Although affording us temporary relief and sometimes even a better perspective on our situation, being sick is usually an unsatisfying way of handling problems. All too often illness itself becomes a bigger problem to manage.

WE USE ILLNESS AS A MEANS OF COPING

"In a culture where feelings are given little importance and emotional needs vital to a person's well-being are frequently ignored, disease can fulfill an important purpose: It can provide a way to meet the needs that a person has not found conscious ways of meeting," we learn from *Getting Well Again*. We cope through illness in part because we are more willing to confront physical problems than emotional ones. Emotional reactions are uncomfortable for most of us, and even distasteful or overwhelming. We scare ourselves by equating great emotional stress and trauma with mental illness, which is so frightening and unacceptable to most of us that physical adversity is more tolerable and easier to confront. We seek help more easily when physically unwell than when struggling with an emotional problem or a difficult circumstance. If we could choose between the two, most likely we would rather be physically ill, but we rarely make such a choice consciously.

Illness may be the only legitimate excuse for missing a day of work or to get the time and space we need for resolving problems, difficulties, or stress. Too often we are expected to return to our everyday routines regardless of personal circumstances like grief, loss, or traumas. Although illness is a socially acceptable way of getting the attention we need, it is also self-defeating for us to have to get sick to get free of obligations, to get time to relax, or to be nurtured.

We often feel powerless and out of control in confronting our symptoms. When they function improperly, our bodies may become a source of bewilderment to us. Illness is one of those circumstance where we ask the futile question, "Why me?" We torture ourselves with questions and blame that further stress our bodies. Our body problems, like ill health, disease, or injury, can also be an arena for drama, for aggrandizing or exaggerating our plight in life, and we can turn an illness into a "soap opera."

COPING WITH PHYSICAL PROBLEMS

Our power exists in how we confront distressing events like illness. We can empower ourselves when confronted by illness by dealing with it directly rather than denying or resisting it. Instead of fighting against it, the secret of coping with physical problems is in letting a symptom or an illness just be exactly as it is. Facing it directly, we can also then take whatever measures are necessary to heal and to heal more quickly. If we discover a sore throat, instead of worrying or denying, we can realize and accept it and then take lozenges or rest or gargle or whatever works to heal ourselves. We are so prone to fighting or questioning, dramatizing or avoiding, that for many of us tolerating, let alone allowing, our symptoms may take a great deal of discipline. We may need to keep reminding ourselves to let go of our worry or upsetting emotions, and especially not to project our worry into the future. If we can accept this body reaction exactly as it is, we then can trust that in this way we will know what to do to best take care of ourselves and heal.

TECHNIQUES FOR EXPLORING PHYSICAL SYMPTOMS

Examining a symptom in depth is another useful way of resolving it. A Gestalt therapy technique is to sit down and really pay attention to and experience the symptom. This is best done by giving the troublesome body part or symptom a voice, to ask that part to speak its feelings *aloud*. A sore throat may speak of feeling constricted or sore at someone or something, and the throat may heal when whatever was inexpressible is said. A stomach pain might tell us what it is that we cannot stomach in our lives so that we can then resolve the problem.

If the body part does not speak up spontaneously, and "it" may not out of lack of practice, we can begin by saying aloud to ourselves whatever is the predominant feeling that goes with the symptom, such as "I hurt" or "I ache." Then our body part can express what "it" or, more specifically, what we are hurting about and denying expression. It may take persistence at first for our body to express the problem or feelings in words, but this is a powerful, effective technique for clearing up physical problems.

Since at one time or another we all use our body to express our feelings for us, it is valuable to learn to examine what a specific body part might say, using our common idiom. We may have a stomach ache: We could ask ourselves, what can't we stomach in our lives? With a headache, we could ask, who or what is a pain in the neck to us? What are we heading off or heading into? Are we having trouble getting headed in the right direction? For a backache, we could ask, what do we want to back out of or back off from? What has gotten our back up, that is, made us angry? Sore throats so often represent swallowed or suppressed verbal expression of our feelings that we can ask ourselves, what are we swallowing? Constipation may open the question, what are we afraid to let go of, or what are we hanging on to? Similarly with diarrhea or vomiting we might ask, what are we getting rid of?

Typically we withhold our anger and resentments, since for most people those are the toughest feelings to express. We also swallow hurt, disappointment, and grief. It is not unusual for us to also suppress anxieties, worry, and fear. Our bodies may be the only avenues we have had up to now for expressing or releasing unpleasant or unacceptable reactions. Once we are willing to express these kinds of feelings in words, our bodies will no longer need to express them for us.

Giving ourselves an opportunity to express our swallowed feelings can relieve us and heal our physical complaints. It can also move us to take action in our lives instead of suffering over problems. Expressing ourselves keeps us healthy and speeds up our recovering ourselves when we are sick. So true is this that patients with cancer, heart disease, and other serious illnesses are being trained to fully experience and express formerly unacceptable and suppressed feelings as a primary means of healing themselves.

Another simple technique to stop the illness cycle of coping with problems in our everyday lives, the cycle in which many of us get caught inadvertently, is a written exercise taught to me by Carl and Stephanie Simonton. This is a written exercise so that the information is concrete and in front of us to use.

Exercise for examining illness: Sit down in a quiet place with a pencil and paper. Then ask yourself these two questions, one at a time, and write down five (or more) answers to each question.

What are the contributing factors to this illness?

What are the benefits from this illness?

Do the first question completely and then the second. Be sure to write five separate answers to each question. The most useful answers could be those we have to dig deeply for or the most obvious. After the answers are written, examine them and categorize them as most significant to the least, with "A" designating the most significant, then B, C, and so on for each question.

As an example, you have the flu, and so you write down everything you can think of that is going on that may be contributing factors:

Overwhelmed with new project at work

Husband out-of-town all week

Angry at an insult by a colleague

Car needs a new muffler and no time to do it

Aunt Mary is visiting next week and she is always demanding

Visa bill was double what was expected

Second snow storm in a week

Then rank them to find the most significant factors in this illness. Any of the items on this list could contribute to illness. However, you might discover that the real problem is that Aunt Mary is coming to visit at a time when you cannot give her the attention she needs. Knowing this now, you might cancel the visit or call Aunt Mary to tell her your situation so that she can reconsider her plans or come knowing you won't be as available as usual. Discovering contributing factors, whatever they may be, frees you to deal with the problems that led to the illness or symptoms and will help you heal all the more quickly.

Listing the benefits of this illness and then ranking them in the same manner can also be illuminating. Your list might read as follows:

New project at work now delayed six months
Can stay in bed and read magazines for a few days
Can cancel Aunt Mary's visit
Husband coming home early from business trip
Can avoid colleague that caused upset
Successfully altered diet
Caught up on sleep

In a workshop with the Simontons years ago, I realized that I loved reading magazines but only did so when I was ill. For me a primary benefit of having the flu was that I could get in bed and read magazines. From then on, I included lying down and reading magazines as a part of my daily routine. I never got the flu again.

Through this method we can tap into our inner selves in such a way as to see what we are using illness to avoid, such as a hurt or disappointment, an unpleasant family quarrel, a job problem, or difficulty communicating. We may have great insights about feelings or moments in our lives that were masked earlier, events that had a much more profound impact than we realized. In the Simonton workshop I attended, another psychotherapist discovered that his unexpected heart attack several months earlier was a reaction to a broken engagement to marry. He had suppressed any grief, hurt, or anger at the time, but in the workshop he realized he paid a very high price for his stoicism.

A common precipitant of illness is the feeling of being over-whelmed by having several stressful events to confront at one time. In and of themselves, each may be manageable, but as a group these events may be overpowering. Several kinds of life changes, moves, or upsetting experiences at one time can throw any one of us into sickness. If that happens, we need to be able to separate out and examine each event and then prioritize whatever steps we will need to take to handle each situation. Acting this way can enable us to be in charge of our lives instead of victimized by our circumstances.

The benefits of illness invariably relate to our needs for affection, comfort, tenderness, understanding, and all that being taken care of comprises. As mentioned earlier, because we adults often imagine or act as if we should be finished with any need to be taken care of, we deny our needs for love or nurturing that then only can be met comfortably when we are ill. Since one of the only ways we get to stop is to be ill, another benefit of sickness is time off from our routines and responsibilities. We need time away from daily routines to restimulate or rest ourselves. A change of pace, like mental-health days and adequate vacations, can be a major force in maintaining good health. Then we would not need to get sick to get time out.

This exercise can make our hidden motivations or reactions more available to us. Most often we cause our own ill health when we swallow important feelings and try to hide our deepest concerns from ourselves. We get sick because we will not confront someone or something unpleasant or because we do not want to make some kind of change. In being more aware of our deeper feelings, we can deal directly with whatever is a problem for us, or we can seek the help we may need to do so.

Done seriously, this exercise can offer us valuable insights for managing our lives more successfully. This method can also prevent future illness. For instance, knowing that we become ill after prolonged visits from certain relatives, we might learn to invite guests for shorter time periods or not at all. Seeing that unexpressed anger leads to body rashes, we might be more willing to say, "I'm angry," when the feeling arises. Noticing that we always get sick when we do not take enough time to nourish ourselves, we might learn to take restful or satisfying time off from the usual routine. Not only do we need to be more conscious of taking good care of ourselves, and whatever that entails for us personally, but in our quest for good health we also need to be more forthright in asking for whatever we need from others.

Our bodies and our health can cease to be a source of suffering for us. First of all, we need to have some knowledge of how our bodies work, both when they are well and when they are stressed. In confronting a physical problem, we need to be willing to discover our deeper motivations so that we can resolve the problems that provoked our symptoms. Acknowledging and working with the often delicate and sometimes bewildering interrelationship between our emotions, minds, and bodies, rather than avoiding or denying it, is one route to good health and ultimately to living fulfilled and free of suffering. Accepting, loving, and appreciating our bodies can be an important source of good health and satisfaction. "Good health," as expressed in *Getting Well Again,* "is the result of paying attention to your needs—mental, physical, and emotional—and then translating this awareness into action."

·IV·

HEALING OUR WOUNDS

• 22 •

Forgiving Ourselves and Others

Never does the human soul appear so strong as when it forgoes revenge,
and dares forgive an injury.

E. H. Chapin

The willingness to continuously forgive ourselves and others is a key source of aliveness in life, as well as a powerful route to not suffering. According to the Merriam-Webster Dictionary, forgive means "to pardon," "to absolve," "to give up resentment," and "to grant relief from payment." Unlike overlooking or condoning, forgiveness implies the need to accept that something happened and cannot be undone. Forgiveness is often a shortcut to finishing our unfinished business with one another, to being complete and satisfied. To continually forgive is a beautiful gift—maybe the best gift—to give ourselves and those around us.

Unfortunately, most of us opt to be "right" rather than to forgive. We bear grudges, hold on to past grievances, and criticize, attitudes which add misery, not joy, to our lives. Our vitality and contentment are limited to the degree that we do not ongoingly forgive. When we hold on to previous hurts, misfortunes, angers, or judgments, our attention and our energies are bound up in the past and today is clouded over; forgiveness allows us to release (or let go) and to complete (or put the past away). A powerful illustration of this point was in a recent newspaper article, where a woman said she would forgive the murderer of her son, "As without forgiveness there's no peace."

Although learning forgiveness may be awkward, it is worth it. Forgiveness affords us freedom, peace of mind, vitality, enthusiasm for life, and the ability to live and love wholeheartedly. However, because of our automatic self-righteousness and our holding on to grievances, we may need to learn to forgive over and over again.

Life would be so much more satisfying if we could accept how imperfect all human beings are and allow for our mistakes, even for our sometimes terrible mistakes. Forgiveness demands a deep compassion for all that being human comprises.

WE WOULD RATHER BE RIGHT THAN HAPPY

We hold on to past injustices, sometimes indefinitely, and thus continue suffering as well. Many of us spend years remembering and blaming someone who wronged us. We sustain our outrage or blame and perpetuate our hurt, disappointment, or distrust. This way we make the other person "wrong" or "bad," and ourselves "right" or "good." Unforgiving, we opt for self-righteousness rather than for intimacy and fulfillment. If we doubt this, look at the lifelong grudges many of us carry against our parents.

We are especially self-righteous and unforgiving toward people with whom relationships did not work out, like former spouses. Lana became a barely functioning recluse after her divorce to prove to her husband how he had wronged her by leaving. Matt went to court to obtain custody of his two small children when his wife asked for a divorce. Years later he bragged that he managed to have her declared an incompetent mother because she left him for another man. Both Lana's and Matt's lives are gripped by their sense of being wronged and their lack of forgiveness.

We can be equally self-righteous about our parents or our children. Some parents disown their children because of an imagined infraction or an upsetting incident. They will not forgive a child who did not obey their wishes or took a job or married someone the parents did not favor. There are also children who refuse to speak to their parents again because of hurtful words or actions. The extreme is when we vindictively cut off another person forever. A tragic newspaper story told of a young man who contracted AIDS and died with strangers. His parents refused to see him because they would not forgive him for being homosexual.

Less dramatic but equally draining are what we would consider the inconsequential areas of lacking forgiveness in our daily lives, areas that are so familiar we barely notice them. We hold grudges against a friend or acquaintance, or someone with whom we work or who is in our employ. We resent or sustain anger or judgments against a storekeeper, dry cleaner, physician, teacher, and the like. Rather than speak up and express our disappointment, annoyance, or hurt, we simply cut people out of our lives, sometimes forever. We satisfy our self-righteousness but we also limit our aliveness in this way.

Instead of forgiving, we perpetuate our grievances by remembering and hanging on to some past event or experience. Thus we cement our feelings or judgments and carry them forward in time. We self-righteously elaborate past upsetting events into powerful, remembered stories or dramas in which we are the central character and often the victim.

Our stories last painfully through time, keeping us aggravated and maintaining our sense of powerlessness. We may not even remember now what is standing in the way with people; we just feel detached or uncomfortable in their presence.

THE CONSEQUENCES OF NOT FORGIVING

We pay a very high price, probably daily, for our lack of forgiveness. We are blind to the sometimes dire consequences of blaming and holding grudges, for we become used to being tired, resigned, and separate from other people. We may not notice how much our current relationships are colored by old events or people, or how cut off we are from our enthusiasm for life. The price we pay for having all our energies tied up in past grievances shows up in our lack of vitality, poor health, troubled relationships, discouragement, loneliness, and isolation from one another.

IT IS HARDEST TO FORGIVE OURSELVES

Usually we are most unforgiving with ourselves. We are very hard on ourselves, for we remember and blame ourselves again and again for old mistakes, mishaps, and disappointments. With memories of our failures secretly alive within us, we are subtly drained of confidence and vitality today. This way we keep ourselves miserable.

We are especially hard on ourselves in response to loss. Working with grieving people, I see that not forgiving ourselves, more than anything else, perpetuates grief years after a loss occurs. With the finality of death and no chance to make amends, we torture ourselves over our past actions, our omissions, and our mistakes. Tragically, most of our unfinished business with lost loved ones is related to some minor infraction that we will not forgive. We become obsessed with self-deprecating ideas and "shoulds," like "I should have been less critical" or "more generous" or "more loving."

Walter, who lost his wife in the fiftieth year of their marriage, was distraught because he had told his wife she looked fat the week before she died unexpectedly. Although she died of natural causes, he blamed himself for her death. In the same vein, so often parents who lose a child regret that they set any limits or spoke harshly to that child, as if that had anything to do with the death. Some of us punish ourselves unmercifully for years after a loved one dies over incidents like these. This is no testimony of our love for the dead, just a painful self-torture.

LEARNING TO FORGIVE

Ongoing forgiveness is a good habit to learn, but we may not know how to do so. Primarily, forgiveness takes the willingness to let go and forget for always. We need to be willing to let go of attitudes, opinions, and feelings instead of hanging on to being "right." We need to stop being caught up in our own narrow perspective and start having compassion. We may never "like" the deed that occurred, but we can learn to accept it.

Taking an honest look will probably reveal incidents or qualities in ourselves or others that we find difficult to accept or forgive. Usually we gloss over and ignore how unforgiving we can be, for lack of forgiveness can become an entrenched habit. To break through it, the first step is to tell the truth about how we feel. For those of us who suppress our reactions in order to be "nice" or to "look good," opening up our honest feelings may initially be very uncomfortable. Know there is a great deal of freedom, peace, joy, and vitality available from speaking the truth. Next are some exercises to open us to forgiveness. These are so valuable that I encourage each of us to stop and do them as soon as possible.

Telling the truth in order to forgive: We should make a list of all the important people with whom we interact—our parents, siblings, children, spouse, boss, co-workers, friends, other relatives—including our own name at the top of the list, with space to write between each name. We need to stop at each name and ask ourselves, "Is there anything I cannot forgive in our relationship?" If there is not, we should congratulate ourselves for that and then go on to the next name. If there is, write it down. Write all of it down—whatever the incident, feelings, and attitudes. We may have a lot written down when we finish this exercise.

Now that we see what we have not forgiven, we should go over each item and ask ourselves if we are willing to accept whatever occurred and to now forgive and forget. If we can just let it go, congratulations! If not, are we willing to have a conversation with that person and communicate responsibly what we have not been willing to forgive up to now? Responsibly communicating would be to say, "I have always felt _____ or I have never gotten over _____ and I want you to know I am sorry I held on to this for so long and I forgive you/me for this." For years I blamed my parents for giving away my dog, a Dalmatian named Chappy. When I finally told them many years later, they immediately defended why they had acted as they did. I didn't want them to feel defensive, so I told them no explanations were necessary. I wanted them to know I harbored these feelings so as to clear up our relationship.

If we cannot speak to the other person—because the person is unavailable or we are unwilling—would we be willing to have an imaginary out-loud dialogue with that person now? As mentioned before, this Gestalt therapy technique of speaking our feelings aloud as if in the presence of another is a powerful tool for completing unfinished business. We can speak aloud to a chair representing the person, or a friend who is representing the person and sitting in to hear our communication. I notice that people often feel self-conscious speaking to an empty chair, so this exercise may be easier to do if we use a friend to represent the person with whom we wish to communicate. Whichever way we do this, complete with the words, "I forgive you, and I forgive me." If these words don't ring true, we should go on. We are not finished yet. When we can freely experience "I forgive you," we have done so.

Once we are free of past grievances, we will need to be vigilant not to create more incidents that we do not forgive. Living in a state of forgiveness is rare for most of us, but it can be done. We will always have reactions to people and circumstances, but our power is in how quickly we can let go of these reactions. Learning to forgive ourselves and others ongoingly frees up our lives and relationships.

Ongoingly forgiving ourselves: To alter our relationship with ourselves, we need to catch ourselves any time we speak ill of ourselves. When we hear a self-belittling statement or complaint against ourselves, right then we need to ask, "Can I forgive myself for that?" If we can, we should do so immediately, speaking simple words like "I forgive myself once and for all for _____." Speaking aloud adds emphasis and makes our words real for us.

The implication is that we are forgiving ourselves forever. That means that at any future time if we have a similar negative thought or a recurrence of this unforgiving idea, we cannot indulge in it. We must remember that we already forgave ourselves once and for all. This is a discipline to be learned over time, so we need to be compassionate with awkwardness and failures as we learn to forgive ourselves.

If we find we cannot forgive ourselves right now, then we need to clear up whatever needs to be said or done in order to be absolved. If "stuck" in unwillingness, we need to ask ourselves, "How long do I need to do penance for that particular misdeed or mistake?" or "How long must I suffer?" or "If not now, when will I forgive myself?" We need to know what steps or actions we must take in order to be absolved or complete. Since we are always our own judge and jury anyway, here is a chance to consciously set our own "penance."

Often clients are unwilling to forgive their loss of temper, their mistreatment of someone, or their inability to cope well with a problem. One woman couldn't tolerate her mismanagement of money; another hated herself for allowing a man to continually hurt her. One man blamed himself for his excess weight, and one couldn't stand himself for alienating his son. Each of these people needed to create a step-by-step plan to come to terms with forgiving themselves, and each of them did.

We can see how exacting and tough we are with ourselves. Thus once we are willing to forgive ourselves, we must act. We have undoubtedly suffered long enough. We usually wait much too long to forgive, and by then we have already self-righteously extracted too much of our own vitality, confidence, and satisfaction. Seeing the price we pay, is it ever worth it not to forgive?

Forgiveness in our intimate relationships: This same exercise of asking what would it take to forgive can be done in regard to other people as well. How long must they pay for their errors? Besides learning to forgive ourselves, the other critical area where we need to learn to forgive is in our intimate relationships. We are as exacting with our intimates as we are with ourselves. Not that we don't each make mistakes, but we don't forget them. Many marriages are stalemated or deadened because one partner or the other cannot forgive an earlier "infraction" or error. A spouse forgets a birthday or copes poorly or acts temperamental or errs, and we remember it always. We tend to think of our spouses with their list of mistakes tacked onto them: This is no longer my husband, but "my husband who earns too little money," or "my husband who embarrassed me," or "my husband who comes home late and doesn't call." This is no longer my wife, but "my wife who yelled at me," or "my wife who spends too much money," or "my wife who dented my car."

Marriages have trouble surviving when one or both of the partners harbor a lot that is unforgiven. Consequently, the habit of forgiveness is especially useful for promoting and enriching our intimate relationships. First off we need to allow that we are human and every one of us makes mistakes. Then we need to plan some time together on a regular basis to clear up anything that needs to be said about our mistakes, anything that is unforgiven. We could take an hour every week or even time each day to express any thoughts or feelings that are harbored. Each person needs to have the freedom to speak, and each needs to willingly listen without judgment, defensiveness, or reaction. It takes big people to be willing to generate this kind of forgiveness together, and these are also the people who have great relationships and lots of satisfaction in life. (In this regard, we might review the discussion of speaking responsibly in chapter 14, "Withholding Ourselves.")

LIVING IN A CONTINUAL STATE OF FORGIVENESS

Our freedom from suffering would expand immeasurably if we could learn to live in a continuous state of forgiveness with ourselves and those around us. Since it is likely that we will always make mistakes, it would help for us to learn to quickly forgive and forget. How satisfying our relationships could be if we were always willing to forgive!

Mastering forgiveness takes awareness and time, even daily, to forgive everyone who comes to mind, past or present, and to forgive ourselves every mistake, flaw, grudge, guilty feeling, or negative thought. We can do it! We can remind ourselves by practicing saying words of forgiveness aloud and with feeling over and over, such as "I forgive myself. I forgive others. I am forgiven."

Remember, forgiveness is the most powerful tool we have for transforming ourselves and our lives. Many of us have experienced that kind of transformation. Years after the fact, I forgave myself for surviving when my brother had died, and I experienced a new freedom and zest for living, a zest that has lasted now for many years. My clients have had similar break-throughs. When Malcolm forgave his mother for never talking about his dead father, he found himself being more powerful and effective in every area of his life. He attributed a subsequent promotion at work to his forgiveness. Nancy's forgiving her abusive father enabled her to at last love herself as well as others. When Enid forgave her husband of twenty years for an infidelity years before, it was as if she had fallen in love with him for the very first time. Their marriage has never been better. This possibility is available for each of us: Let's forgive ourselves and everyone else around us for anything and everything, for therein lies the promise of a rich and satisfying life.

• 23 •

COMPLETING OUR EXPERIENCES

What a wonderful life I've had! I only wish I'd realized it sooner.

COLETTE

As suggested throughout this book, being complete promises an end to the common, everyday suffering we all experience; it is one of the great secrets of being satisfied in life. Complete means "over" or "ended," encompassing what in Gestalt therapy is called finishing our "unfinished business," which entails letting go of the past, be it a past event, feeling, memory, or person. To be complete means to be whole or perfect, to have no part lacking, and it also means to be fully realized. Complete, we are free to be alive and present to life right now, free of the past and open to possibility and challenge.

Life is more of an ordeal when we drag our unfinished business around with us. Finishing unfinished business is the process of letting go of or releasing something or someone, out of which we experience freedom, relief, extra energy, and openness to new possibilities. Although we may have to move through some intense or difficult emotions or get there, ultimately completing is satisfying.

Probably we all have a great deal of unfinished business in our lives. Most of us live with long written or unwritten "to do" lists that we do not complete, lots of clutter, and lots of history that we continually drag into the present. Our inner state of disorder is reflected in our living with excess things and situations around us that are old, unwanted, and unexamined, all of which keep us feeling depleted and muddled.

Although we may not be aware of it, our incompletions drain us. They hang around in the background of our lives all the time, waiting, pulling at our energy. The converse, finishing our unfinished business, then can potentially give us a lot of extra energy to invest in life. Both the act of completing something and the increased energy resulting from that act can generate added satisfaction and room to create newly.

We tend to enshrine in our memory and hang on to almost everything that ever happens to us, especially past hurts, traumas, and disappointments. Most of us resist completing things. We are blind to the fact that we habitually carry around a great deal of both internal and external old and excess baggage that drains our lives. Even though learning to be complete with our experiences and our history is critical to mastering life, it is not something most of us do naturally.

Our suppression of ourselves, regardless of our rationale for doing so, invariably leaves us with a great deal of unfinished business. Most of us walk around suffering with strong feelings and thoughts that we never express, reactions that neither disappear nor cease for us. We either consciously withhold ourselves out of our idea of being "nice" or appropriate, or, more insidiously, we swallow our feelings and reactions automatically without realizing it. Thus incomplete, we are apt to live halfheartedly, stifled, enervated, and tired, and we become so used to it that we may not realize that life could be any different for us.

EFFECTIVE ROUTES TO COMPLETION

Declaration: Taking the stand that we are complete and living our lives accordingly can be very effective. We declare we are complete regardless of our reactions or circumstances, and out of this stand we let go once and for all of our positions, feelings, attitudes, or ideas. It is over. Once our thoughts, memories, or feelings from the past are declared complete, there is no room for us to indulge in rehashing them. Our promise to be complete empowers us to stop anytime we catch ourselves reopening what we already declared to be complete. If we are committed to keeping our word, our promise or declaration keeps us on track.

This kind of stand taking can be particularly valuable in the area of managing suffering, as described in chapter 5, "The Commitment Not to Suffer." We can choose or commit ourselves not to continue to grieve or hurt, to limit the amount of misery we suffer. This was evident to me in letting go of both my parents, for either of these losses could have been debilitating for me. If I dredged it up, I could find some upsetting memory or issue. Long relationships are bound to have some unfinished business. Yet, taking the stand that I was complete with my mother and father freed me to say good-bye to them right away, freed me to go on with my life, unhampered by regret or suffering.

We can elect not to suffer over a divorce, or a loss, or an illness, or a disappointment. We can literally take charge of how much pain we endure, and we can choose when to stop agonizing. The dignity and power and aliveness that we feel when we commit ourselves to such a stand can enhance our lives incredibly. Taking charge this way, the past is left in the past and today is open and free.

Fully reexperiencing the incompleted past event or relationship: This is the second, more elaborate method of completion. This technique requires our fully experiencing all of our emotions or reactions, forgiving ourselves or others, and then saying "good-bye."

Mostly we stay attached to past upsetting events and carry them around because we do not know what to do with them. Developing this skill in completing would help us deal with all kinds of experiences, upsets, and traumas and would free us to live more present to and alive to today.

Margaret healed a major trauma in a two-hour therapy session with me using this "finishing" technique. She came to me to complete with a tragedy that occurred five years earlier. Traveling in a foreign country, she and many others were injured in a train derailment. Margaret was now filled with tension and fear and was "going through the motions of living," and she dated this shift in herself to the train accident.

I asked Margaret to tell me the story of the accident in detail, encouraging her to literally relive it exactly as she remembered it moment to moment. As she related the details, intense emotions emerged. She felt fear, anguish, and particularly grief at all the dead bodies she remembered. I had her stay with this moment for a long time, describing all the details, so she would fully experience all of her formerly suppressed emotions. She cried as if the accident were happening now.

Margaret's attention kept returning to the dead children lying outside the train, which for her was the heart of the trauma. She couldn't bear what she saw. That's what made her cry the most. As if in passing, she mentioned her own extensive injuries, the many broken bones and painful bruises over her entire body. Only when I pressed for details did she elaborate about herself, for her total attention was focused on how the accident affected others. Help was slow in coming, but Margaret convinced a passerby to take her in his taxi to a medical center miles away. She spent months healing in a hospital far from her home.

In continuing to explore Margaret's story, I realized that the obvious trauma of what she saw and felt, her body injuries, and her long recuperation away from home were not the heart of what was keeping her riveted in the past and incomplete now. She seemed to have come to terms with all of these aspects of the accident. What eventually emerged was the guilt that she had suppressed until then, guilt that she had survived and so many others had not. What has left a lot of room for Margaret's guilt is that she could not help the children.

Margaret was ridden with guilt because she sought help, was taken to a fine medical center, and survived the accident. She was sure that everyone else died at the accident or later from poor medical care. Her completion work involved her grieving and saying "good-bye" to all the dead people from the accident. Most crucial was Margaret's forgiving herself for seeking help, which she had thought "selfish," and for not helping others.

In traumatic life events, like Margaret's, our greatest anguish may be that we are the ones who survived. Being a survivor of a war or an accident often generates a particular kind of personal torture, for seeming to be singled out to live can be very disturbing and bewildering. Much more attention is being given today to the special trauma of being a survivor, and these experiences, too, can and need to be completed.

Margaret's memory of her experience was vivid. However, sometimes old memories can be vague. Often what we are dealing with in past experiences is what we imagined and not necessarily what actually happened. That does not matter.

Whatever we are suffering over is what needs to be completed, whether factual or not.

Margaret's experience demonstrates that we can be complete with anything that happens to us. Our willingness to be complete is the single most important step to doing so. Sometimes we unknowingly set a specific, prescribed time that we think necessary for our suffering. Then we won't be open to completing upsetting events until we have done the appropriate "penance" that we set up for ourselves, perhaps unconsciously. We need to uncover and review our ideas or beliefs about "penance," for what we demand of ourselves may be harsh and inhibiting.

Earlier we examined the human penchant for storytelling and dramatizing and how it deflects the truth. Used for the purpose of completion, however, storytelling has a different significance, since it can bring us closer to our own, often hidden, personal truth. The critical distinction is in the purpose of our relating our experience as a story. When we tell the story of our lives to get attention, to exaggerate our misery, or to gain a similar "pay off," there is no change of being finished with the experience. However, reliving our story in order to finish with it is very beneficial.

In completing, we tell the story but once in full detail, wherein we can reexperience all the emotions, thoughts, attitudes, and beliefs that are tied up in this event. At this time we can fully grieve and express our feelings, forgive ourselves and others, and say good-bye forever to whatever or whoever caused us pain. We can be complete through the full expression and release of all our emotions and attitudes and memories.

Gestalt therapy "finishing" technique: This is the same technique used earlier for letting go of parents. We need to either select a listener we trust to sit and listen through this process with us, or, if we have the courage, we can go through the process alone. Either way, we will need a chair or pillow in front of us to represent the person or trauma or event that we intend to complete or finish. We will then talk *aloud* to the event or person.

We should begin by stating what happened and then allow and express whatever feelings come up—hurt, anger, disappointment, regret, longing, shame, or any other feelings. Although there may be several kinds of feelings, probably one emotion will predominate. Beliefs or thoughts may arise as well—like Margaret thinking that she was somehow responsible for saving the other people in the accident. These are details that hold the story or the pain in place, and yet the details are not as crucial as the feelings.

The key is getting in touch with the suppressed emotions that keep this incident or experience painfully alive. Once expressed, we will feel lighter or freer or more relaxed, and so we need to stay with our feelings until there is the sense of that kind of release. Next, we need to stop and forgive the situation or person or forgive ourselves aloud. We would then say good-bye aloud to the person or event that has caused so much pain. This good-bye is not just words but really a commitment to have the event or memory or trauma over once and for all—right now.

WHAT IT IS TO BE COMPLETE

How do we know if we are complete? Even though the upsetting incident is probably not forgotten, now there is a lack of intense feelings or "charge" around that memory or event. Lack of "charge" is the clearest indicator of being complete.

We may also notice a sense of relief or peacefulness or disinterest concerning what was formerly turbulent for us. We can remember without distress. We may respond to formerly charged events in new ways, or we may not react at all to situations or people that once were stirring for us. We can know we are complete by the ease with which we confront someone or something formerly difficult to confront.

Complete with our lives, we live now from moment to moment with no attention on the past or the future. We are satisfied with whatever this day holds rather than preoccupied with what has been or what should be or what is missing now. We live life directly as it is happening, not as a memory or a longing, alive to or on the edge of every new moment. We appreciate the delicacies of life, the scenery around us, that loveliness of intimate moments, the wisdom in ourselves. We are free.

When we are complete, we are not torn by "if only"s or hurts or disappointments. We do not bemoan our fate or wait endlessly for life to turn out as we would like it to. We are too busy living to worry, doubt, blame, or regret. When we are complete it is evident that we are truly the source of our own satisfactions, the creators of our lives. Our relationship with ourselves can also be vastly different once we are complete, for most of us are such habitual fault-finders and self-torturers that it would be extraordinary for us to accept ourselves exactly as we are now.

Complete with ourselves, we are open to love, intimacy, and enrichment in our relationships with other people. Instead of living separated and distrustful, at loggerheads with one another or in a sullen but polite armed truce, we can fully enjoy and appreciate one another. We are free to be with people as they are instead of always longing for them to fit our pictures or ideals. We can love others, even on a global scale.

It has been stressed throughout this book that we live most satisfied whenever we are complete with ourselves, other people, and the past. Completion can be accomplished by a stand that we take on our lives, a no-matter-what commitment that we are complete, or by specific techniques to finish, express, and relieve our unfinished business. Although the process of completion can be awkward to learn, challenging, and even rigorous, the results are well worth it. By being complete, we have the chance to have a truly full, unlimited life.

• 24 •

RECOVERING OURSELVES: TOOLS FOR HEALING

Life is like playing a violin in public
and learning the instrument as one goes on.

SAMUEL BUTLER

O nly in fairy tales does the hero slay the dragon once and for all and live happily ever after. In real life the dragons keep coming. Considering the dragons we will probably have to slay in a lifetime, each of us needs to have an ability to recover ourselves. Since the course of life rarely runs smoothly, we need tools for handling our inevitable encounters with life. Unfortunately for most of us, how we recover is often a hit or miss affair. Because we tend to deny that life can be confrontational, we do not necessarily learn to expand our coping skills to use again.

WE CAN LEARN TO HEAL QUICKLY AND EASILY

Our attitudes about our own healing are critical to the outcome. If we believe we have to take a long time to recover, invariably we make that a fact. If we believe we can recover easily in a short period of time, we tend to do exactly that. Most important, if we think we have no power over the outcome, we will make that true as well. Our beliefs and intentions very much affect the speed at and the means through which we recover.

Changes in life can shake us to the core, at least for the moment. When shaken, we need to be able to stop and allow ourselves some peace and quiet and ease to heal ourselves. We are usually more sensitive to this need when ill or physically injured and less sensitive to injuries to our psyche, heart, or soul. Too often we pay no attention to a possible psychic trauma, so that we intensify our stress by trying to pretend life is as usual.

We need time to heal, but we do not need forever or even years to recover from life's events. Life is too short for that. We may be able to recover ourselves in days or weeks if we are committed to healing as quickly as we appropriately can. The speed with which I get through losses, disappointments, upsets, and pain matters to me, for in the past I took fourteen years to mourn my brother's death. I know how debilitating and unhealthy such extended recovery periods are.

Unless the event that befalls us is a monumental trauma like the death of a loved one or disaster, we are often blind to our recovery needs. We can have strong reactions to events like job losses, bankruptcy, illness, or caring for a sick relative, and to major life moves like marrying, having a child, having a child leave home, or changing jobs. Stress symptoms can include lack of energy, sleeping more or less than usual, physical symptoms, or depression.

The process of healing ourselves, how long it takes, and how we recover is an individual matter. Remembering how we sustained and healed ourselves in the past can help us recover now, so it is useful to list recovery tools that we can then call upon when necessary. Listed below are some specific guidelines for recovering and healing ourselves during or after a crisis. These are suggestions, not requirements, and are not a "to-do" list with which to add stress to our lives, but we can benefit from taking action in each of the areas mentioned.

TOOLS FOR HEALING

1. Diet: A healthy, well-balanced diet of proteins, vegetables, fruits, grains, and a minimum of fats and sugars aids our healing. We need to educate ourselves about what comprises a healthy diet; that information is available from our physician, the American Heart Association, or other health groups. It is useful to know that too much sugar depletes us and to discover which foods energize us.

2. Exercise: Regular exercise like walking, running, swimming, bicycling, playing tennis or racquetball, and so on at least three times a week is also helpful. While a person is either under stress or recovering, I recommend daily exercise as is appropriate for the individual, for anywhere from twenty minutes to two hours, to increase his or her energy and sense of well-being. This can particularly make a difference after a loss, trauma, or stress.

3. Rest: In contrast to activity, we may also need rest. Those of us who tend to drive ourselves hard may recover best with rest periods, lying down and taking it easy sometime during the day. "Cat naps" or reading breaks or closing our eyes for fifteen minutes can be rejuvenating. Both rest and sleep can regenerate us.

4. Meditation: This is another form of rest or rejuvenation. Taking twenty minutes one to three times a day to go

inward can be very healing since daily quiet time can help us relax and regenerate ourselves. There are many techniques for and books on meditation. One simple form of meditating is to sit with closed eyes while listening to classical music for twenty minutes.

5. People Support: Daily support of a friend, colleague, therapist, counselor, teacher, minister, or rabbi is valuable nourishment. We benefit when we can talk intimately, clear up feelings and reactions, be understood, or have a witness to our experience, and be encouraged to move forward. Friends and family may worry too much about us or get too involved in our problems or be unavailable, so at times someone outside our regular life can be the most supportive of our recovering.

6. Nourishment: Activities that nurture our bodies, like massages, hot baths, sun baths, or whatever personally appeals to us, are particularly supportive. The kind of nourishment I am speaking of is not related to eating and food. Many of us habitually deny our needs, so we may have to dig deeply to discover what would nourish us. We can uncover our needs by examining what the contributing factors to our current stress were, using the exercise described in chapter 21, "Our Bodies and Our Health."

7. Time Alone: In my experience real healing often necessitates that we take time alone to do nothing, to look at the scenery, to read, to daydream, to watch television, and particularly to rest. How much time alone each of us spends may vary. I take time by myself every day, and I notice that my spirituality and creativity emerge during or after the time I spend alone.

8. Time Off: Time away from our routine, a contrast to the every day, like vacations or days away from home, can also be effective. If vacations are not feasible, consider a drive or walk in the country or any environment different from the usual. Since I lived in a beautiful countrified area, for me nourishing time away may mean going to a place like San Francisco or New York for more excitement.

9. Play: Playing one hour a day can be regenerating. Many of us lost the idea of play as we grew into adulthood. We may need to look newly at what play would involve for us now—games, sports, shopping, or crossword puzzles are a few examples of what we might enjoy. It is startling yet true that as adults we do not generally have much fun.

TAKING RESPONSIBILITY FOR OUR OWN RECOVERY

After reading through the suggested tools for healing, we should make a list of the specific steps that would help us heal or recover. What do we find relaxing, delighting, engaging, or fun? Having written all these answers down for further use, we can carry them in our daily calendars or post them on our mirrors or refrigerators. We now have some practical, hands-on ways of generating our own healing.

• 25 •

RECOVERING CONFIDENCE AND A SENSE OF SELF

*The most vulnerable and at the same time the most
unconquerable thing is human self-love; indeed,
it is through being wounded that its power grows
and can, in the end, become tremendous.*

NIETZCHE

A kind of recovery of which we may not ordinarily be aware
is recovering our sense of ourselves, the regaining of our
confidence, courage, willingness, sense of purpose, or whatever
quality we lack that is preventing us from feeling whole and satisfied. This kind of healing does not necessarily occur naturally and
may demand specific actions on our part.

To recover ourselves we need to be aware that something is
missing. We may notice that we lack confidence or that we are
living halfheartedly all of a sudden. Although we may not know
the source, we usually notice when we have a persisting drop in
confidence or enthusiasm or a loss of affinity with ourselves or
others. These are times when we need tools to literally recover
ourselves.

Reconnecting with loving ourselves is the key to this kind of
recovery. Although "love thyself" may sound like a cliché, few

of us put this maxim, which is essential to our well-being, into practice. We need the support of our own love most of all. For whether we realize it or not, we are the most important person in the world for ourselves. Chances are that all of us could use help generating self-love. Some never learned how and some mock the idea as a negative expression of the "Me Generation." Nevertheless, none of us can thrive without our own love, appreciation, and respect.

AN EXERCISE IN LOVING OURSELVES: THE MIRROR TRICK

A powerful technique for reconnecting with loving ourselves is to stand and face ourselves in a mirror and to say aloud, "I love you. I need you. I value you. You are the most important person in the world to me. I cannot make it without you." This is a potent way to reaffirm our relationship with ourselves. Notice the results. Doing this exercise regularly will remind us that we are committed to a partnership with ourselves. Another way to use the mirror daily is for each of us to look at ourselves and say, "I love you exactly the way you are." These are probably the most effective words we could ever speak to ourselves.

Being compassionate with ourselves is an important aspect of self-love that can deeply influence how we feel and how we function. We might recover immediately if we would just pay loving attention to ourselves. However, we are more apt to develop our criticizing muscle. We learn to observe and destroy, to dissect and dislike, to scrutinize and judge. Our training in self-criticism is deeply ingrained. To counteract what I call our "critic," we need to work at developing our compassion-ate side, which is often like an undeveloped or unused muscle. To teach self-love, I devised Self-Compassion Lessons for my clients. Just as some of us went to dancing school as children to learn poise, grace, and good manners, we could also benefit from training courses in loving and accepting ourselves early on in life.

TREATING OURSELVES COMPASSIONATELY

We can have an impact on our sense of worth by treating ourselves in a new way. We can learn to stop and ask ourselves the questions we wish someone else cared enough to ask us, like "What's wrong?" or "How are you doing right now?" or "What would you like to tell me?" or "How can I help?" Even though it has unfortunately become another cliché, it is deeply rewarding to act as our own best friend.

Observing ourselves with compassion: We may be compassionate toward other people, yet few of us love or accept ourselves just as we are. The way I teach compassion is by having the client pull up a third chair next to me, and look with me at the place where they were formerly sitting. I suggest they observe themselves as I have done, free of judgment. I ask what they see, and I coach them to notice their pain or difficulty or admirable qualities in a loving, sympathetic way.

Sometimes I enlist my client to be my co-therapist or consultant as a structure for being supportive of themselves. I may talk about them caringly, such as, "Look how hard Mary is struggling over this. How could we help make it easier for her?" Or "Mary is being so hard on herself. What could we say to help her feel better about herself right now?" We are so often kinder to ourselves acting as a third person in this way than we ever are on our private stage.

Being compassionate by being your own therapist: We need to have a way of developing compassion on our own when there is no one to model ourselves after. Use two chairs, one entitled "the compassionate seat," from which you will observe "yourself" in the other chair. As in the session described earlier, take time to notice and express aloud your appreciations of you. Speak aloud in an understanding way about the problems or attitudes with which you are currently struggling, talking with yourself as if you are a friend or counselor who has your best interests at heart.

From this new vantage point, you can begin to view yourself with more concern, understanding, and lovingness. You can truly shift your relationship with yourself by doing this exercise regularly.

MASTERING COMPASSION

Few of us speak well of ourselves. If we listened intently, we would hear how often we speak derogatorily and disparagingly of ourselves. Usually we view ourselves with a critical eye that is quick to pick up our flaws or mistakes. We are often disconcerted or embarrassed by our own humanness.

Speaking well of ourselves as a daily practice: Practice is the road to mastery. Because we are more in the habit of speaking negatively, complaining, and downgrading ourselves, shifting will take real vigilance and practice. We need to begin to listen to exactly what words we say when we speak about ourselves. Listening newly, we may hear ourselves automatically saying things like "I'm not good at that," or "I screwed up again, just like always," or "I'm such a clod." **STOP!** These are occasions when we can alter our words on the spot to learn to accept and appreciate ourselves. "I am good at that" or "I am graceful or capable" would be much more supportive. We might transform our lives if we spoke well of ourselves.

Acknowledging ourselves as a daily practice: In addition to compassion, acknowledgment boosts our self-esteem and enables us to recover ourselves. We all need to be reminded that we did a job well, or spoke clearly, or appeared handsomely, or achieved our goals, or that we are good persons. Acknowledging ourselves daily is a good habit to adopt, for it will have a powerful impact on how we live. Some of us still have the old false idea that compliments and acknowledgment lead to conceit and arrogance. Not true. When we are respected and appreciated, most of us flourish and grow. However, since the world is not generous with its acknowledgments of us, we must fill that gap ourselves.

AN ACKNOWLEDGMENT EXERCISE

Structuring time for compassion helps to establish it in our awareness. Set aside two or three time periods a day for personal appreciation. Times connected with other regular habits like meal times, teeth brushing, or physical exercise help us be faithful to this retraining of ourselves. We are particularly vulnerable to self-deprecation just after we wake up in the morning and before we fall asleep at night, so both are opportune moments to do this exercise. During those periods set aside for acknowledgment, we can run through the day's events moment by moment, acknowledging everything and anything good about ourselves.

A SECOND ACKNOWLEDGMENT EXERCISE

Another way to use the time we set aside is to list ten successes each day or say ten positive things about ourselves. We acknowledge waking up on time, not picking a fight, getting a piece of work done, looking attractive, and keeping our word about doing this exercise. We can appreciate qualities like our perseverance or lovingness or grace under pressure, and ultimately we can learn to appreciate whatever we see in ourselves.

Instead of glossing over or ignoring lapses in our compassion for ourselves, we can view them as opportunities for acknowledgment. Once we move away from habitual criticisms, eventually we will have a natural, well-deserved, and deepened respect for and acceptance of ourselves.

Appreciating what we have or are instead of complaining about what we do not have enhances our sense of ourselves. Most of us want what we do not or cannot have, and so we miss enjoying what is available for us right now. We can be so much happier if we accept and appreciate however life is right now. The most important stand we can take on our lives is to say, **"What I have is more important than what I do not have."**

• 26 •

RECOVERING BY CONTRIBUTING TO OTHERS: THE SUREST MEANS OF HEALING OURSELVES

The only gift is a portion of thyself.
RALPH WALDO EMERSON

Every one of us cares that our life matters or makes some kind of difference, and we can ensure that we make a difference by serving other people. Our lives then mean something. Nothing I know of makes a greater impact on our self-esteem than this. Contributing to other people is a potent secret for healing, feeling good about ourselves, and for having a life worth living. Whether we give ourselves to individuals or to the world at large, in serving others we discover or recapture the best that we are. We experience our largeness, breadth, and depth, beyond our small concerns or complaints.

Also, in a very practical sense, making ourselves available to assist others and having our attention off ourselves can generate change and growth and a sense of personal power and effectiveness within us. For many years I have been active in the hospice movement in this country and have seen how many of the most effective volunteers are individuals who themselves had suffered major personal losses. Involving themselves with other people's grief was a critical part of the volunteers' recovery, for making a difference in the lives of others nourished and healed them. This same holds true for people who are active in organizations for AIDS patients, cancer recovery groups, and Alcoholics Anonymous, to name a few. Engaging ourselves with other people's problems can free us from our concern with our own.

The power of service has shown up many times in my own life. Once I took a volunteer job of registering 250 people for a workshop, which fortuitously occurred the day after a major love relationship ended. I cried all day, and with some irritation pulled myself together to do the promised volunteer work that evening. For five hours I was involved with all those people, their paperwork, their concerns and needs. For those five hours I truly forgot that my relationship had ended, as I was so focused on the needs of the workshop participants. The discovery that I could literally put my own grief aside for the sake of other people was a great gift to me. It gave me this critical information: We do not need to suffer twenty-four hours a day over any problems or upsets, not even over our most major tragedies. I also saw that a most potent way to free oneself of pain is to be fully engaged in giving to other people.

The value of serving the world was most articulately expressed by George Bernard Shaw in *Man and Superman*:

"This is the true joy in life, the being used for a purpose recognized by yourself as a mighty one, the being a force of nature, instead of a feverish, selfish clod of ailments and grievances complaining that the world will not devote itself to making you happy. I am of the opinion that my life belongs to the whole community and as long as I live it is my privilege to do for it whatever I can. I want to be thoroughly used up when I die. For the harder I work, the more I live. I rejoice in life for its own sake. Life is no brief candle to me. It is a sort of splendid torch which I've got a hold of for the moment and I want to make it burn as brightly as possible before handing it on to future generations."

Because life hurts, we will always need to be able to heal from both physical and emotional pain. We must recover our sense of ourselves at any given time, so that we can be fully engaged in life and continue to live with vitality and satisfaction. We have now looked at many different means of nourishing ourselves and recovering that affect both our attitudes and beliefs. Above all, service is one of the most effective strategies for feeling well and living well. Nothing makes us stronger than realizing we make a difference. Living with purpose will be discussed in the next chapter.

• 27 •

RECOVERING BY STRUCTURING OUR LIVES WITH PURPOSE

The people who get on in this world are the people
who get up and look for the circumstances they want,
and, if they can't find them, make them.

GEORGE BERNARD SHAW

Living based on a purpose is life-affirming and renewing. A purpose can help us find the courage to go on, no matter what problems we confront, and the courage to combat despair or discouragement. Any new step—a commitment, goal, hobby, friend, plan, or interest—can make a difference and can reawaken us to purposeful living apart from our pain. Thus, actualizing a simple plan to learn a new subject or quit smoking or keep a journal or build a bookcase can turn our lives around.

If we are to live as designers instead of as victims of our lives, we must keep generating something to live for. What impelled us yesterday may not exactly fit today. We need to review and revise our commitments to keep life fresh, alive, spontaneous, and satisfying, since without purpose we may feel lost or despairing. Continually creating goals with more goals behind them enlivens us.

A purpose that is large enough can inspire us for an entire lifetime. An implicit problem here is that some people wait around endlessly for the "right" purpose to show up, and it doesn't. Purpose is something we have to generate for ourselves. Hence, we would be wise to simply make up a purpose from which to live, and then commit ourselves to it. Our purpose could be a big one: to end war or hunger on the planet or to love every other being in our world. However, our purpose does not have to be a lofty one to be satisfying, for any new step can make a difference in regenerating our vitality and satisfaction.

At different times I have struggled to find meaning and something to make life worth living. For many months, writing this book and the anticipated completion of it were powerful daily inspirations, something worth getting up for every morning that also made tomorrow enticing. The possibility of touching people and releasing them from suffering has given me an enormous sense of purpose. All through my life I have seen that aspiring to contribute to others, more than anything else I do, gives my life meaning or purpose. We all need to look for what inspires us.

There are many kinds of purposes that can inspire our lives. A mother raising healthy, happy children has an involving purpose, as does a child completing a complex science project. A woman or man who runs or works out in a gym daily to keep fit or who operates an impeccable office are living from purpose. The person who drives a bus loaded with handicapped children to school has as great a purpose as the person who manages to maintain a clean environment. Determined, conscious living that leads people to feel satisfied and enlivened by a job well done, whatever that job may be, is what it means to live from purpose.

Life would be more satisfying for most of us if it were supported by any purpose that we deem worthwhile. It usually doesn't work to have another person be our only purpose in life, but there are times when we may give all of our attention to a relative or friend in need. When all our energies are tied up with just one other person—a spouse, child, lover, or parent—we are apt to end up feeling depleted or deprived. Most of us need more in order to feel satisfied. Also, people are transitory, while a purpose, if large enough, can inspire us indefinitely.

RECOVERING THROUGH HAVING COMMITMENTS

Specific promises that we keep can make a major difference in our feeling good about ourselves and our lives. This is one way we can surely strengthen and support ourselves. Notice how much satisfaction we feel when we can commit to being on time or keep our word or when we stay on a diet or complete a piece of work. This holds true of any promises or commitments we make and keep.

Giving our word in any area of our life can make a real difference in how we feel about ourselves and our lives. We can promise to take care of ourselves in some way—dieting, exercising, or having fun—and thus enhance our lives. Promising to work out a particular relationship problem can transform a relationship. If we promise to stop getting angry or criticizing, or if we promise to stop taking someone else's lateness or silence as a personal attack, or if we promise to give more or to ask for more, we can truly alter our relationships with one another. Likewise, we can have an impact on our work life by making promises to complete work or to start new projects or to behave in some new or more effective way. Making and keeping a promise in any area can enhance our daily lives immeasurably.

As a busy psychotherapist, I made a commitment to write a minimum of seven hours each week and to exercise four times a week. Then I planned my life in such a way that I kept my word to myself to do these tasks faithfully. No matter what my mood or what distractions occurred, my promise served as a guideline to keep me on course. An exciting bonus derived from keeping my promise was this book, which I began writing with no plan, no outline, and no design ahead of time.

MAKING PROMISES

These ideas may inspire us to stop, consider, and then make our own list of what promises would enhance our lives. We could write down where and how we would like to alter our lives. Use the following list of powerful commitments as a guideline. This can be useful for generating any kind of commitment that would inspire and expand us. Our list of promises can represent how we would like to live from now on.

LIST OF PROMISES

I am committed to forgiving myself continuously.
I am committed to letting go of the past.
I am committed to letting go of grief.
I am committed to acknowledging myself every day.
I am committed to living effortlessly.
I am committed to contributing 100 percent of myself.

I am committed to having exciting work.
I am committed to having an exciting relationship.
I am committed to having a healthy body.
I am committed to celebrate life and to laugh.

This is not a frivolous exercise to do and then forget, for it has great power for altering or transforming our lives. Therefore, after our commitments are established, it helps to make them concrete by posting them in visible places. This way we will be reminded often of how we choose to live our lives.

We can commit ourselves to having our lives be great! Promises, tailored to our own needs or interests, can expand our satisfaction, stretch us, and be our personal standard for living successfully. Keeping our commitments supports us to live as the designer instead of the victim of our lives. Not only can we generate renewed zest for life with promises, but we can also overcome anything that befalls us by committing ourselves to recovering from it.

• 28 •

THE SECRETS OF SHORTCUTTING HURT

> *Do not wish to be anything but what you are,*
> *and try to be that perfectly.*
>
> ST. FRANCIS DE SALES

This chapter is a summary of some of what it takes to overcome hurt and suffering. The most important element in overcoming the pains and crises of life is the willingness to take on the challenge that life is, instead of being a victim of your experiences. Next, you need to be conscious enough that you do not keep putting salt into your own wounds by dramatizing or personalizing, by living in the past, by being right about suffering, and by withholding yourself. Finally, you need to be willing to be complete with your experiences and to forgive and forget.

The following are the basic steps to shortcutting life's hurts. First, you need to be present to the experience of pain or of any other feelings at the moment when they occur. Then, you need to fully express all the related feelings and reactions. Next, you need to be willing to overcome these feelings or this experience and even to commit yourself to do so. Finally, you need to let go or forgive and forget as soon as possible to free yourself to go on with your life. There is no way you can end up feeling like a victim of your experiences, if you manage them with this kind of awareness of what it takes to recover and heal.

Being present to your experience, whatever it is, means just that—living your experience as it happens, confronting the moment head-on instead of running away or distracting yourself or closing down. When something traumatic or shocking occurs, you may initially feel numb and lost. You may feel fear or nausea or anger. You may wish you were a thousand miles away from this moment. It is important that you notice and allow each of these responses as they occur, for noticing and allowing your experience is part of staying with it. Being present does not necessarily involve action so much as your willingness to allow and stay with what is happening right now.

There are times when, in order to be present, it may also mean going to wherever you are needed, or calling, or, as a last resort, writing a letter. If someone else needs your help or is in pain, don't hesitate to go there if you can, to give solace or love or physical assistance. This can be a satisfying opportunity to contribute to another and to heal yourself, as well as a chance to complete with that person or situation and to say good-bye. If you are intent on being complete with your experiences, you will invariably know what you need to do to accomplish completion.

It is very important that you always make sure you have the occasion and a safe place to express all of your feelings and reactions as soon as you can. Tell a friend, family member, or a counselor, but do not miss an opportunity to cry or say whatever it is you are feeling. Speak aloud your hurts or fears, your regrets or angers, and speak now, not waiting for next week or some seemingly better time. The Kahuna saying, "Now is the moment of power," is apropos here. Expressing yourself fully and freely, you can release—perhaps forever—all that is connected with this painful moment—now.

Be committed and willing to overcome whatever you are experiencing, whether you are facing an illness, a loss, a disturbing event, or whatever. That will give you a sense of power over your circumstances and will help you surmount whatever you have to confront. Remember that there is enormous power in taking the stand of "I will" or "I can." Even if you don't believe these words right now, by starting to use them you can turn your life around.

Next you must be willing to let go of your pain and go on. It is your choice to let go of pain or not. You are not a victim, for you can choose how and how much you suffer. It is essential, then, that you examine any beliefs or ideas or history that keep you from being willing to heal today.

Learning to forgive and forget is essential. You may have little experience in this realm, but many tools for accomplishing these feats are elaborated on throughout this book. Especially see chapters 22 and 23 on forgiveness and completion. Remembering pain keeps it alive, perpetuates it.

Forgive and forget everything from the past, so that you are free to be fully alive today. Complete everything. Forget the source of the pain, for it really doesn't matter anymore. It is never too late to forgive or to say goodbye to experiences or events or people from the past. Say whatever you need to say and do whatever you need to do, but be sure you have no unfinished business with the past. In so doing, you will give yourself the enormous freedom to live fully present to today, and the possibility of living a great life.

• 29 •

LIFE IS A GIFT

*It's a funny thing about life: If you refuse to accept
anything but the very best you will very often get it.*

W. SOMERSET MAUGHAM

Every one of us wants to make our life work, but this often turns into a frustrating project of trying to control the uncontrollable. We think to be in charge of our lives we need to control our world, and then we suffer in frustration and perhaps despair. The unsuccessful behaviors we have examined, like being right about suffering, living in the past or the future instead of in the present, searching for meaning where none exists, or being "loners" in life, all represent the fallacy that we can somehow control life.

In truth, how much control have we had over our lives so far? Life is full of unexpected events, changes, losses, and ordeals beyond our control. We are doomed to suffer if all our attention is on trying to control what is not in our power to control. Instead, we will have so much more power over and satisfaction with our lives if we are open and awake to life's possibilities. For whatever way we choose to confront it, life is sure to be full of surprises at every turn.

One of the special secrets of having a life that is satisfying and easy is this: **appreciate life instead of resisting it**. Appreciation is the ability to get outside of our reactions, story, concepts, and beliefs in order to see the beauty, the value, and the preciousness of life. Appreciation is gratitude for life. We fully appreciate life when we can see the wonder of it all.

As children we naturally appreciate and value everything we see. We can be awed by a set of keys, a baby goat, or assorted pots and pans. We delight in all of it. As experience intervenes, we discover hurt, disappointment, and failure. Then we lose our sense of wonder, so our capacity to see and appreciate narrows. Life intrudes until wonderment and openness are virtually replaced by cynicism and resignation. Once our wonderment disappears, we forget that there is anything for which to be thankful.

In learning to manage the forces around us, we let go of the wonder of life. We become intent on developing survival skills instead of stopping to appreciate the flowers or to love one another. In our drive for control, we forget pleasure and joy and satisfaction. Even though we will always wish we could control life, we do not have to be run by these survival tactics. We can choose our responses to life. We can choose to have life be an energizing and provocative challenge that we take on powerfully rather than a series of ordeals of which we are victims.

To demonstrate this choice of how we view our lives, the old story of the optimist and the pessimist is appropriate here. Two children are each given ponies for their birthdays. The optimist is delighted by and appreciative of the gift she receives. She cannot wait to ride her pony. She is full of all the choices, all the possibilities of life now that she has her own pony. The pessimist is not happy, for he sees how much work the pony will be, how costly the pony's food will be, and how much manure there will be to clean up. The pessimist cannot enjoy his pony.

This story illuminates an important message: Satisfaction is not necessarily found in our circumstances. It is not what happens in our lives as much as how we perceive what happens and how we live through what happens. How we view our lives and the events that occur is what makes all the difference in the quality that life has for us. The pessimist tortures himself, and the optimist is delighted by and appreciative of the gift he receives. This can be true with each and every moment or event in our lives—will we appreciate it or be disappointed?

Each one of us has an opportunity to choose how we will view all the experience in our lives. We can choose to see our lives and each and every event in our lives as a gift! Imagine what life could be if we were delighted by and appreciative of everything that happens to us, every human encounter, every mood change, and every kind of event that occurs. We would not then judge events or people as good or bad, as pleasant or unpleasant, as wanted or unwanted. We would appreciate *all* of it.

Imagine how powerful it could be to see the opportunity in a loss, the opportunity to feel deeply, to have known such love or the opportunity to learn to let go, to pick ourselves up and begin life newly, differently than before, or the opportunity to feel compassion for someone else who hurts. Imagine seeing a loss of a home or a fire, as Sara did, as an opportunity to get rid of history, to start life fresh and new. Imagine living through a divorce as a chance to start over, no longer influenced by a partner. Imagine choosing to complete a relationship with dignity instead of hatred. Imagine taking on life with new vigor or in a new way after an illness or an accident. Imagine choosing to stop suffering. NOW!

Appreciating all of life, we can see painful events as opportunities, for those are the moments that truly stretch us and expand us to grow and deepen beyond who we think ourselves to be. In what may seem the worst of times, when we face loss and death and tragedy, we discover our heroism, our courage, our love, our creativity, and our power. These seemingly catastrophic experiences are occasions to stretch ourselves beyond whoever we have been up to now, to play life full-out. They are profound challenges.

Real life hurts and disappoints. However, out of our willingness to live a real life, instead of trying to force life to fit our unrealistic pictures, we can expand and grow beyond our wildest dreams. In reviewing my life, I see so clearly that the many painful experiences in my life have been gifts, for each was an opportunity for me to grow bigger, stronger, and surer of myself. Each allowed me to have a deeper understanding of and compassion for myself and for other human beings. Each led me to a new possibility and a greater depth. I am sitting here today at peace with all of it. The opportunity in life is to accept ALL of it. Yes, life hurts, but the pain does not last, especially if we are truly committed to letting go of suffering. Begin today.

I hope that now you can include pain and suffering as part of human experience and not be overwhelmed by the likelihood that sometimes life will hurt. The willingness to be open and awake to life, to engage wholeheartedly in life, and to live with passion means that you will reach enormous depths and expanses of human experience. And sometimes life will hurt. But know that you have what it takes to recover yourself quickly. You don't have to suffer. NOW ENJOY YOURSELF!

ACKNOWLEDGMENTS

Thank you to all my friends and clients who have shared their lives with me, for through this book your experiences will inspire many other people. Special thanks to my agent and friend, Jed Mattes. At HarperCollins, I thank Larry Ashmead for his friendship and his faith in me and my work, and Janet Goldstein for being a truly brilliant and inspiring editor. Special thanks to my friend, Gregg Stebben, and to Cory Allyn at Skyhorse Publishing for making this new edition of *You Don't Have to Suffer* possible.

INDEX

ABOUT THE AUTHOR

Judy Tatelbaum, LCSW, is a psychotherapist, public speaker, and author of the best-selling book, *The Courage to Grieve* (HarperCollins, Inc. 1980), and video/CD *The Courage to Grieve, The Courage to Grow*. She grew up in Rochester, New York, graduated from Syracuse University, and has a Master's degree from Simmons College School of Social Work. A foremost authority on overcoming emotional suffering, grief, and other life crises, she is committed to encouraging people to face and recover from adversity, and to showing people new possibilities for creating satisfying lives. Because of her inspiring stand for people, she is a popular professional speaker and trainer. She lives with her husband in Carmel, California.

Her website is: www.JudyTatelbaum.com

You Don't Have to Suffer is a book that is used by
psychotherapists and medical personnel; cancer, AIDS,
hospice and bereavement groups and staff; clergy;
health and psychology courses in colleges and universities;
libraries; students; teachers; and the general public.
Judy welcomes comments and stories from readers
about the impact of reading this book.
Her email is: Judy@JudyTatelbaum.com